LIFESTYLE
PLAN

THE INVALUABLE STUDY GUIDE TO
MAXIMIZE THE BENEFITS OF...

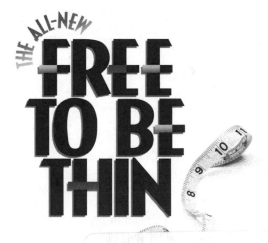

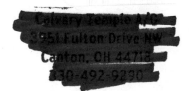

Books by Neva Coyle

Abiding Study Guide
Daily Thoughts on Living Free
Diligence Study Guide
Discipline Study Guide
Discipline tape album (4 cassettes) with guide
Free to Be Thin, The All-New (with Marie Chapian)
Free to Be Thin Lifestyle Plan, The All-New
Free to Be Thin Cookbook
Free to Be Thin Daily Planner
Free to Dream
Freedom Study Guide
Getting Your Family on Your Side (with David Dixon)
Learning to Know God
Living Free
Living Free Seminar Study Guide
Making Sense of Pain and Struggle
Meeting the Challenges of Change
A New Heart . . . A New Start
Obedience Study Guide
Overcoming the Dieting Dilemma
Perseverance Study Guide
Restoration Study Guide
Slimming Down and Growing Up (with Marie Chapian)
There's More to Being Thin Than Being Thin (with Marie Chapian)

LIFESTYLE·PLAN

THE INVALUABLE STUDY GUIDE TO MAXIMIZE THE BENEFITS OF...

THE ALL-NEW FREE TO BE THIN

·NEVA COYLE·

BETHANY PUBLISHERS HOUSE
Minneapolis, MN 55438

Published by Bethany House Publishers
A Ministry of Bethany Fellowship, Inc.
11300 Hampshire Avenue South
Minneapolis, Minnesota 55438

Printed in the United States of America

Library of Congress Cataloging-in-Publication Data

Coyle, Neva, 1943–
    The all-new free to be thin lifestyle plan / Neva Coyle
        p. cm. — Personal journal and study guide for use with The
all-new free to be thin.
    1. Reducing—Religious aspects. 2. Christian life—1960–
3. Reducing—Study guides.
I. Chapian, Marie. Free to be thin. II. Title.
RM222.2.C44   1993 Suppl.
613.2'5—dc20   93–25601
ISBN 1–55661–343–1   CIP

This personal journal must be dedicated to the many thousands of Overeaters Victorious members who have written to me expressing their thanks, reporting their victories, and sharing their struggles. Because of their encouragement, I've had the courage to continue looking for answers when I wanted to give in to discouragement and give up. I dedicate this book also to the many hundreds of Overeaters Victorious group leaders whom I've never even met—those who on their own initiative have taken up the ministry in their local churches or groups and carried this network of encouragement into places I could never go.

Finally, this journal is dedicated as well to the OV board of directors who have served unselfishly and given of themselves to encourage me and hold me accountable.

NEVA COYLE is Founder of Overeaters Victorious and President of Neva Coyle Ministries. Presently she is the Coordinator of Departmental Ministries in her church. Her ministry is enhanced by her bestselling books, tapes, as well as by her being a gifted motivational speaker/teacher. Neva and her husband make their home in California.

She may be contacted at:

P.O. Box 2330
Orange, CA 92669

A NOTE FROM NEVA

I'm glad you've chosen to turn to the Lord for help with the problem of overweight or overeating. I'm also glad you've chosen this biblically-based program as a means of seeking His help. Here you'll find exceptional insights and encouragement for dealing with the perplexing challenges you face.

In the fifteen years since the original *Free to Be Thin* was written, much more research on overeating and overweight has been completed, and more information has been gathered. As these more recent findings have become available, I've made a special effort to keep up-to-date and to present them to those involved in the ministry of Overeaters Victorious through books and other literature. This new information is reflected in this study as well as in the revised version of my book *The All-New Free to Be Thin*.

Recent research reflects positive changes in our culture's attitudes toward those who are overweight. At the same time, however, even stronger warnings have been issued about the dangers of overeating and the importance of healthful food choices. Both the new attitudes and warnings should be of importance to those of us determined to please God in every area of our lives, including the stewardship of our bodies.

My prayer is that as you complete this study, you'll be changed—not just physically, but emotionally and spiritually as well.

Because of Jesus,
Neva

Acknowledgments

A special acknowledgement goes to Bethany House Publishers, especially to Carol Johnson and to Jeanne Mikkelson, who have stood by me through the years. They believed that there was always an important lesson to be learned in all my struggles, and that those struggles could help many others through the printed word.

CONTENTS

FREE TO BE THIN—
WHAT'S IT ALL ABOUT?

The National Center for Health Statistics says 16% of Americans are 30% or more over desirable weight (1983 statistics). Women are more likely than men to be at the extremes of either under- or overweight.

According to the 107th Annual Statistical Abstract of the U.S. Census Bureau, the average woman in the United States today is 5 feet, 4 inches tall and weighs 142 pounds—a little heavier than ten years ago. The average male is 5 feet, 9½ inches tall and weighs in at 173 pounds—slightly less than a decade ago.

Studies also surprisingly reveal that approximately one third of American women are above the size 16 range, creating an unprecedented market for today's "women's" fashions.

In 1988 Americans spent an estimated $10 billion and more on weight-related products and programs. Obesity research costs $24 million or more annually.

We now know that 31% of all American women between the ages of 19 and 39 diet at least once a month. Even though over 70 million of us dieted in 1988, only 1 in 10 was able to keep that lost weight off for any length of time. The sad truth is that almost 95% of those who lose weight will put the weight back on—plus more within 2 to 5 years.

Our culture, while promoting thinness, is producing fatness. Our American fascination with convenience has encouraged a diet with over 40% of its calories coming from fat.

We're a culture of vast contradiction. While living a fat lifestyle, our children, many as young as the age of 6, have already formed prejudices against overweight people. Youngsters go on self-prescribed diets as early as eight or nine years of age—many beginning a long and even deadly battle against weight cycling, eating disorders, and a distorted sense of body image and self-worth.

11

A long-held belief in our society is that overeating is the fundamental cause of overweight. Yet studies are now showing that overweight can be caused by many factors. No one factor at work in an individual's life can make a person fat without the complex interaction of many other factors. Overeating can be and is a key factor in many cases, but so are genetics, dieting history, weight-loss cycling, and much more.

Since overeating is so commonly the cause of overweight, the first part of this program will target eating habits. Some who complete this program—maybe even you—will discover that when principles of discipline are applied to eating habits, weight will come down. But others will not find this to be true. If overeating is not the cause of your overweight, this journal will lay that accusation to rest once and for all.

Our first series of lessons will address your weight problem as if it were simply caused by overeating, despite the strong probability that other factors are involved. As we move on to other subjects of study, along with new eating habits, emotional issues that can also affect your weight will be discovered and confronted. We hope that bringing several factors together will help you find some answers for your particular weight problem.

We take a unique and biblical approach to the problem of being overweight. This is not simply another diet group—it's a ministry of hope, acceptance, understanding, and love. Get ready for a change!

OUR FOCUS

The focus of this study is not weight loss, but ministry to overweight people and overeaters. We emphasize changed habits and attitudes leading to a deeper relationship with Jesus Christ.

This approach is totally new—it even differs somewhat from the earlier methods of Overeaters Victorious. Please don't be in a hurry. Rather, take pleasure in developing new disciplines and focusing on inner change, not just on outward appearance or adherence to a set of rules. Give yourself time and be patient with your progress. Remember these words of Scripture: "He who began a good work in you will perfect it until the day of Christ Jesus" (Phil. 1:6, NASB).

God is willing to take all the time necessary to do a work only He can do.

OUR HISTORY

Overeaters Victorious (OV) began in 1977, when two friends and I met in a private home to offer mutual support while looking deeply into what God's Word had to say about overeating and weight loss. All three of us were struggling with discouragement about the failure of weight-loss programs. From that small beginning came the approach now known worldwide as *Free to Be Thin*.

My two friends eventually dropped out, but I became increasingly interested in the problems facing the overweight Christian. I continued my study, keeping detailed records of my discoveries and thoughts. From those notes came the entire Overeaters Victorious program.

My own continuing struggle with weight management has kept me sensitive and realistic in my expectations for "thinness." I know and understand the needs of the overweight Christian probably as well as anyone else around. I never refer to overweight people as *them*, but always as *us*.

OV has outgrown the earlier concept of a formal program, and become a more broad approach now used in churches, small informal settings, and by individuals. We've tried to make this personal journal and leader's notes as easy to use as possible, without requiring formal ties to an organization or leadership training.

OUR PROCEDURES

The OV strategy is simple. First, each day—preferably in the morning—read the Scripture text assigned on the Daily Journal Sheet and respond in the spaces provided. At each day's end write your thoughts in the space for reflections. At the end of the week, or before your class or group meets, answer the questions for that lesson and complete the weekly evaluation. Our food plan is based on the widely accepted exchange program of the American Dietetic Association.

Exercise is a critical part of our program. We'll introduce it early at beginning levels to make it easier to incorporate into your daily life.

Our Goal

The goal of this book is best expressed in the words of Susan Wooley, Ph.D., Co-director of the Eating Disorders Clinic and Associate Professor of Psychiatry at the Cincinnati Medical College:

> ... to help [overweight people] come to some kind of lasting and permanent resolution of the weight issue. To find a weight they can accept, that they can live with and get off this bandwagon once and for all. And to try to return to them some sense of dignity, self-respect, and control.

Your Group Leader

If you're using this material in a group, no doubt the leader of your group will be a great resource for you in the days to come. A willingness to help you when you need it, a determination to hold you accountable when necessary, and a commitment to pray for you regularly have been the common characteristics of all the Overeaters Victorious group leaders I've ever met. They've also demonstrated a special love and acceptance for group members, which have rapidly become the trademarks of Overeaters Victorious all over the world.

Nevertheless, your success in this program does not depend solely on your group leader. It depends on *you* and the commitment you make to put into practice the things you'll be learning.

How to Use This Book

1. This book is arranged for use over thirteen weeks. It will fit into the quarterly system of a church program, or it can be used individually, or in a small group of friends.

2. The sections called "Preparation for Lesson . . ." include each week's instructions. They may vary, so be sure to read them every week.

3. The food plan will be introduced in Lesson Three and can also be found in Appendix E.

4. The textbook for this study is *The All-New Free to Be Thin*, and I include a reading assignment at the end of every lesson-preparation section. Please read the book as you use this journal. Become familiar with it, and keep it handy as a manual and reference book while you daily walk out your new lifestyle.

5. A section called "Group Guideline Suggestions and Leader's Notes" begins on page 243.

6. As an added help, try the *Free to Be Thin Food Supplement* flip-style calendar. This handy little item can provide just the right word of encouragement as you go about your daily routine. Many of the thoughts for the day used in this personal journal are from that calendar and are used by permission of the publisher (published by Garborg's and available through your local Christian bookstore).

From my own experience, I can assure you that you're on the threshold of a miracle in your life—a miracle beyond anything you could ask or think!

MY GOALS FOR THIS STUDY

Please provide the following information before you begin this study.

I need to make improvements in the following:
- ☑ attitudes toward myself
- ☑ food habits and choices
- ☑ a consistent exercise routine
- ☑ a daily quiet time
- ☑ attitudes toward others

I have the following prayer needs: _____
_____
_____
_____

Other comments: _____
_____
_____
_____

Other goals: _____
_____
_____
_____
_____

My weight today: _____ Date: _____

My eating habits are
- ☐ out of control
- ☐ somewhat out of control
- ☐ controlled but with some periods out of control
- ☐ careless
- ☐ a little careless
- ☐ sometimes careless, but sometimes quite rigid and controlled

I find myself
- ☐ totally giving up on disciplined eating
- ☐ going between extremes of disciplined and undisciplined eating
- ☐ wanting discipline and consistency, but realizing that I need help and support.

A BOLD NEW BEGINNING

Whether you're a new Free to Be Thin class member or a former Free to Be Thinner, this study is for you. If you're stuck on a plateau, have stopped trying, or have regained weight, this study has been written with your needs in mind. If you find yourself lacking in enthusiasm, this study promises you a fresh start. The Scripture readings included in this first week offer wonderful promises of renewal.

First, follow the Bible study closely on days one to five and receive these beautiful promises from God. On day six, do the lesson. On days six and seven, try walking in the new truths you've learned—without leaning on the paperwork. You may find that freedom scary at first, but accept God's grace in trial and error.

Second, keep in mind that this approach is new! It offers new attitudes, new disciplines, new fresh words from our Father just for you, right now.

Third, for now, don't count calories. Calorie guidelines will be given later, but for now, this is the beginning of a renewed obedience of the heart.

Fourth, enjoy liberal doses of the "Food Supplements" (listed in Appendix A page 257) several times a day. Whenever you feel hungry, experience the temptation to overeat, or feel the urge to eat at all, grab this book and turn to the "Food Supplement" section. Pour them into your spirit in massive doses. Read them aloud through gritted teeth or tears, if necessary. Force-feed your spirit on them as you pull the flesh back into control. These "Food Supplements" are perfectly safe—you can't possibly overdose on them.

Fifth, identify what you understand to be sensible and healthful eating patterns. Address between-meal and bedtime snacking habits. Make an effort to "search and replace"—that is, spot those eating habits you already know aren't healthful and wise, and ask God to help you replace them with other choices, such as fresh fruit or vegetables, or with foodless activities.

Most important: Get the promises of the Scriptures in this first week's journal pages deep into your spirit so that all outer change comes from inner change through the Word of God.

✔ Read *The All-New Free to Be Thin*—Chapters 1–2.

GOALS FOR THIS WEEK:

- To have a daily quiet time using the Scripture readings assigned.
- To recognize changes I need to make in
  - food choices
  - attitudes
  - other: _to get started_
- To identify which items I can replace with healthier choices.
- Other goals:

_____

_____

_____

DAY ONE   **READ ISAIAH 43:18-19**

GOD IS DOING A NEW THING!

God is impressing on me that . . .

I've shared with the Lord that . . .

Thought for the Day:

It's new, it's now—there's no better time to begin a bold new walk of obedience.

Today's Challenge:

Beginning your first new day means you're on your way. What new thing do you anticipate God doing in you?

Food Diary	Present habit:	Replace with:

God is impressing on me that . . .

I've shared with the Lord that . . .

Thought for the Day:

Doing things God's way will take patience on your part. God is not on your schedule; make it your purpose to be on His.

Today's Challenge:

Cultivate the desire to do God's will.

Food Diary	Present habit:	Replace with:

God is impressing on me that . . .

I've shared with the Lord that . . .

Thought for the Day:

An undivided heart is a heart already turned toward obedience. It makes decision-making time so much easier.

Today's Challenge:

I will maintain a heart attitude in keeping with God's will for me.

Food Diary	Present habit:	Replace with:

DAY FOUR

READ PSALM 28:7-8

HE WILL STRENGTHEN YOU AND SHIELD YOU.

God is impressing on me that . . .

I've shared with the Lord that . . .

Thought for the Day:

When faced with temptation, it's better to trust in the Lord for strength than to try to resist on your own.

Today's Challenge:

Will you completely trust the Lord today? How do you anticipate His helping you?

Food Diary	Present habit:	Replace with:

A NEW YOU!

God is impressing on me that . . .

I've shared with the Lord that . . .

Thought for the Day:

When God makes a change, everyone who sees it, knows it.

Today's Challenge:

Today I will settle the following issues:

Food Diary	Present habit:	Replace with:

A BOLD NEW BEGINNING

There comes a time in each of our lives when a prolonged struggle of some sort leaves us desperately declaring, "Enough is enough!" The parable of the Parodigal Son (Luke 15:11–32) tells about just such a time in the life of a young man. He had strayed so far from his wealthy father that he was reduced to slopping hogs just to be able to share their food. That frustrated youth, too, decided that enough was enough.

Desperate situations call for daring decisions, and boldness to take the first steps necessary for a solution and freedom. For example, despite his embarrassment and fear, that young man took action when he said, "I will arise and go to my father," then set out for home. We too must take the same kind of bold first steps.

This is the time. There is no better time than now to begin the bold new experience of a walk of obedience to God. And just as the young man of Jesus' parable found his father waiting, we will find our Father God waiting. His arms and His heart are open.

This week's Scripture readings are promises of a new beginning. The last reading also promises that God is willing to act on our behalf. "I will do it," says the Lord. Will you let Him?

In your own words, write your thoughts about "Our Focus" on page 12:

_____
_____
_____
_____

When God does something new, it's not like anything we've ever experienced before. If He were to do something totally new in you in the following areas, how do you think you would change?

- eating habits

_____

_____

_____

_____

- attitude about my weight

_____

_____

_____

_____

- attitude toward other overweight people

_____

_____

_____

_____

- attitude toward thin people

_____

_____

_____

_____

What new principles has the Lord taught you this week?

_____

_____

_____

_____

How could you be more faithful in honoring the Lord next week?

_____

_____

_____

_____

What was your favorite "Food Supplement" this week, and why?

_____

_____

WEEKLY EVALUATION

Goals for the week that I have seen realized:

_____

_____

_____

Goals that were set but only partially realized:

_____

_____

_____

Goals I will carry over to next week because they are worthwhile and important to me:

_____

_____

_____

Goals that I will drop or adjust because they were unrealistic or unimportant:

_____

_____

The most important thing I learned from this week's lesson:

_____

_____

_____

A victory I would like to record:

_____

_____

_____

I am surrendering to God . . .

_____

_____

_____

I am choosing to be more obedient to God in . . .

_____

_____

_____

PREPARATION FOR LESSON TWO

WE REALLY DO NEED ONE ANOTHER

1. *Write*

Before you begin this week's preparation and lesson, fill in the questionnaire on page 261 (Appendix B), and keep it in mind when following the quiet time guide and the lesson questions. If you're meeting in a group, bring it with you to the next meeting.

2. *Daily quiet time*

Using the guide on the following pages, read the assigned Scripture texts for your daily quiet time and use the provided spaces to note your responses.

3. *Read*

If you can, review *Getting Your Family on Your Side* by Neva Coyle and Dr. David Dixon (Bethany House Publishers, 1987).

4. *Ask yourself*

In Appendix C, there are some questions you must carefully and prayerfully consider. Read them several times and then answer in the column as indicated.

5. *Prayer partner*

In Appendix D is a special promise to a prayer partner. Begin now to ask God to provide just the right partner in prayer for you. Also pray that He'll make you into the right kind of partner.

6. *Food plan*

Maintain what you understand to be a sensible eating plan but with this one change: Modify your daily food intake to include as many as five or six servings of fresh fruit and vegetables.

✔ Read *The All-New Free to Be Thin*—Chapter 18.

Goals for This Week:

- To have a daily quiet time using the Scripture readings assigned.
- To recognize changes I need to make in
  - _____
  - _____
  - _____
- Other goals:

_____
_____
_____
_____

DAY ONE   **READ ECCLESIASTES 4:9–12**

WE REALLY DO NEED ONE ANOTHER.

God is impressing on me that . . .

I've shared with the Lord that . . .

Thought for the Day:

Our job is not to straighten one another out, but to help one another up.

Today's Challenge:

I will let myself need someone today by . . .

Food Diary	Prayer Partner Possibilities 1. 2. 3.
	A victory I had today
Total Fruit & Vegetable Servings:	

God is impressing on me that . . .

I've shared with the Lord that . . .

Thought for the Day:

Being a team player isn't as much a matter of vulnerability as it is humility. Could it be we hide behind our pride and disguise it as a need or as a fear of being hurt, when the truth is that we really believe others don't matter?

Today's Challenge:

To be a good prayer partner I will change:
1.
2.
3.

Food Diary	Prayer Partner Possibilities 1. 2. 3.
	A victory I had today
Total Fruit & Vegetable Servings:	

God is impressing on me that . . .

I've shared with the Lord that . . .

Thought for the Day:

It's not that we *have* a part in the body of Christ—but that we *are* a part of His body.

Today's Challenge:

I will show an interest in the function of others in the body of Christ.

Food Diary	Prayer Partner Possibilities 1. 2. 3.
	A victory I had today
Total Fruit & Vegetable Servings:	

PUT UP NO STUMBLING BLOCK.

God is impressing on me that . . .

I've shared with the Lord that . . .

Thought for the Day:

Do I have the love and strength of character to surrender food choices that would discourage another person from doing his or her best?

Today's Challenge:

I will encourage someone else in the realm of food choices.

Food Diary	Prayer Partner Possibilities 1. 2. 3.
	A victory I had today
Total Fruit & Vegetable Servings:	

God is impressing on me that . . .

I've shared with the Lord that . . .

Thought for the Day:

When we encourage one another, prefer one another, and live in unity we strengthen one another—all the while witnessing to the world of Christ.

Today's Challenge:

I decide to change my attitude toward relationships in the following ways:

Food Diary	Prayer Partner Possibilities 1. 2. 3.
	A victory I had today
Total Fruit & Vegetable Servings:	

LESSON TWO

WE REALLY DO NEED ONE ANOTHER

After completing part one of the questionnaire in Appendix B on page 261, what new insights do you have about yourself and your weight-loss history?

_____

_____

_____

_____

After completing part two of the questionnaire, page 262, what new insights do you have about your emotions and overeating?

_____

_____

_____

If you are married, based on your answers to part three of the questionnaire, page 263, is your spouse more likely to be a supporter or a saboteur? Explain.

_____

_____

_____

Based on the promise to an OV partner in Appendix D, page 267, what kind of partner do you think you need?

_____

_____

_____

_____

What kind of partner do you think you can be?

_____

_____

_____

_____

Why do you think you're ready to go on to the full "All-New Free to Be Thin Lifestyle Plan?"

_____

_____

_____

_____

A SPECIAL NOTE

Our hope is that you have family support, and at least one friend in addition to your OV partner who will be of help to you during this time. If you do not have this kind of support, knowing where your support will *not* be coming from will help when others unknowingly or carelessly sabotage your plans.

Thousands of Christians are studying this material, walking in new truths, and finding strength in Jesus Christ right now—along with you. People who don't know your name are praying for you each day. Won't you do the same for OVers everywhere? We really do need one another—to love, accept, and pray for one another each day.

Weekly Evaluation

Goals for the week that I have seen realized:
_____
_____
_____

Goals that were set but only partially realized:
_____
_____
_____

Goals I will carry over to next week because they are worthwhile and important to me:
_____
_____
_____

Goals that I will drop or adjust because they were unrealistic or unimportant:
_____
_____

The most important thing I learned from this week's lesson:
_____
_____
_____

A victory I would like to record:
_____
_____
_____

I am surrendering to God . . .
_____
_____
_____

I am choosing to be more obedient to God in . . .
_____
_____
_____

PREPARATION FOR LESSON THREE

FIRST THINGS FIRST

With the foundational insights we've gained from the first two lessons, we're ready to begin in earnest to make changes in our food choices and eating habits. This week we will start to utilize the food program part of the lifestyle plan.

First, we will compute our calorie needs for safe weight loss. This helps us to understand what we are undertaking.

Second, we take this effort to God and make it part of our relationship with Him.

Third, we look at some objectives to help us keep our focus on that relationship while finding strength to carry out our goals for behavioral change.

Computing Calorie Needs

You are unique. Your body is special. You're not exactly like anyone else you know, so you deserve a little individual attention in computing your caloric needs. The following formula will provide you with an individualized guideline to help you achieve your goal of a new healthy lifestyle. Our special thanks goes to Dr. C. Wayne Callaway, nutrition and weight expert, and author of *The Callaway Diet* (Bantam Books, March 1991), for this simple, personalized method for determining individual needs.

WOMEN

1. Begin with a base of 655 calories   _____655_____
2. Multiply your weight in pounds×4.3   _____
3. Multiply your height in inches×4.7   _____
4. Add together the totals from #1, #2, and #3   _____
5. Multiply your age×4.7   _____
6. Subtract #5 from #4.

   (This is your normal resting metabolic rate.) _____

49

7. Multiply result of #6×1.1 _____

8. Round off #7 to the nearest 100.
(This last figure is your daily calorie need.) _____

MEN

1. Begin with a base of 66 calories _____66_____

2. Multiply your weight in pounds×6.3 _____

3. Multiply your height in inches×12.7 _____

4. Add together the totals from #1, #2, and #3 _____

5. Multiply your age×6.8 _____

6. Subtract #5 from #4 _____

7. Multiply #6×1.1 _____

8. Round off #7 to nearest 100.
(This last figure is your daily calorie need.) _____

No doubt you are surprised by these calorie limits, because they are higher than the ones most doctors used to recommend. But Dr. Callaway, former director of the Nutrition and Lipid Clinic at Mayo, is joined by many other specialists who now agree that we need to make less drastic cuts in calorie intake so that we give our metabolism time to correct itself.

The American Dietetic Association reports that the new, higher-calorie limits serve four purposes:

1. to keep metabolic rate at a normal level.
2. to keep from losing lean body tissue along with fat.
3. to keep weight losses at modest rates.
4. to keep from setting yourself up for failure and regain.

A summary of the food choices based on the exchange lists provided by the American Dietetic Association is found in Appendix E, page 269. Menu suggestions computed for various calorie limits are included in Appendix F, page 273.

With your calorie needs computed and your food choice guidelines and menu ideas firmly in your mind, now follow the daily quiet-time assignments as you did for Lessons One and Two. Use the Food Diary column as a place to record your food choices and to list their exchange values. At the bottom of the sheet is a place for recording your totals so you can see whether any adjustments are needed.

▶ Read *The All-New Free to Be Thin*—Chapters 3–4.

GOALS FOR THIS WEEK:

- To have a daily quiet time using the Scripture readings assigned.
- To recognize changes I need to make in
  - food choices
  - attitudes
  - other:_____
- To identify which items I can replace with healthier choices.
- Other goals:

_____
_____
_____

God is impressing on me that . . .

I've shared with the Lord that . . .

Thought for the Day:

We don't make a covenant with God. We simply enter the covenant He has proposed to us. That covenant has nothing to do with thinness—but *Lordship*.

Today's Challenge:

I acknowledge God's love for me today and thank Him for it.

Food Choices				How Many?	Exchange Group:

Total Exchanges

Bread	Meat	Vegetable	Fruit	Milk	Fat

God is impressing on me that . . .

I've shared with the Lord that . . .

Thought for the Day:

Just because it's not too difficult doesn't mean it's easy.
Often things within our reach still require us to stretch.

Today's Challenge:

My hope today can be summed up in the following
words:

Food Choices	How Many?	Exchange Group:

Total Exchanges

Bread	Meat	Vegetable	Fruit	Milk	Fat

God is impressing on me that . . .

I've shared with the Lord that . . .

Thought for the Day:

Food choices aren't made in the kitchen, but in the heart.

Today's Challenge:

I plan to make several good choices today, including:

Food Choices	How Many?	Exchange Group:
Total Exchanges		

Bread	Meat	Vegetable	Fruit	Milk	Fat

God is impressing on me that . . .

I've shared with the Lord that . . .

Thought for the Day:

The gift of choice is God-given. It's not the right to do what we want, but the freedom to choose to do what He asks.

Today's Challenge:

I will obey today by . . .

Food Choices	How Many?	Exchange Group:

Total Exchanges

Bread	Meat	Vegetable	Fruit	Milk	Fat

God is impressing on me that . . .

I've shared with the Lord that . . .

Thought for the Day:

I can choose to obey Christ or to follow a program. While the methods may appear to be identical, the motivation is quite different.

Today's Challenge:

I will see all God's children as His and to appreciate them as such.

Food Choices	How Many?	Exchange Group:
Total Exchanges		

Bread	Meat	Vegetable	Fruit	Milk	Fat

Lesson Three

First Things First

Moses, the great leader of God's people, once climbed a mountain to get a closer look at God (see Exodus 19). No doubt that action also gave God a closer look at Moses. On the mountain, God spoke to Moses about entering a covenant of obedience to Him. Only after the people agreed to the covenant did God give the particulars of the law they were to obey, including what we now commonly call the Ten Commandments.

As people under the new covenant of grace given through Christ, we still confuse these two concepts. We mistakenly believe that obeying the commandments is the same as being in covenant with God. But if we look at God's covenant with Moses, we realize that the commandments come *after* the covenant. They are statements of how those who live in covenant with God are to live their lives.

People who live in covenant with God serve only Him. People who live in covenant with Him don't misuse His name. Instead they revere it and hold it precious. They remember to keep a day holy, set apart for Him; and out of respect for how He brought them into being, they honor their parents. They don't kill or harm anyone; they keep themselves pure within the bonds of marriage; they don't steal or lie, nor do they live in envy of another's possessions. A lifestyle, not a set of rules, marks the lives and hearts of God's children.

As you, too, enter this time of covenant with God concerning a change in eating habits and attitudes toward your body, let the covenant—not the rules—be the focus of your response to God.

A covenant with God is not the same as a contract between two people who each agree to live up to their end of the bargain. Rather, a covenant with God is a relationship with Him in which He is the sole provider. He is the Giver and we are the takers. God does have His terms, but they're not so hard that we can't accept them. They only require that we live in obedience to His

62

will and His word and learn to walk in His ways. What's more, it's all in our best interest. But we must remember that there is nothing to negotiate in a covenant with God. We either take His terms or refuse them. It's as simple as that.

In the past several days you've been reading Scripture texts about a covenant relationship with God. These verses state that what He asks of you, while being within reach, will require a walk of obedience. He offers you life-changing choices and a change of heart to become obedient. Will you respond to His call?

God doesn't just give us a set of rules and then step back to watch how many we break. Rather, He offers us a relationship. That covenant relationship is itself the source of our strength to follow simple guidelines, which in turn give us an opportunity to express our covenant relationship with God in the everyday matters of our lives.

A loving God is calling you today to enter a new covenant relationship with Him. How will you respond? Write out your answers to the following questions in the spaces provided:

If I let my relationship with God affect my food choices, how will my eating habits change?

_____

How will *I* change?

_____

What decision will I make now about my covenant relationship with God?

_____

What does each of the following statements mean to me?
• Positive change is a matter of relationship.
• What God is asking of me is not too hard or out of reach.
• My weight or eating problems require a walk of obedience.
• God offers me, not body-altering, but life-changing choices.
• God is calling me to accept a new heart to be obedient.

WEEKLY EVALUATION

Goals for the week that I have seen realized:

_____

_____

_____

Goals that were set but only partially realized:

_____

_____

Goals I will carry over to next week because they are worthwhile and important to me:

_____

_____

_____

Goals that I will drop or adjust because they were unrealistic or unimportant:

_____

_____

The most important thing I learned from this week's lesson:

_____

_____

_____

A victory I would like to record:

_____

_____

_____

I am surrendering to God . . .

_____

_____

I am choosing to be more obedient to God in . . .

_____

_____

_____

PREPARATION FOR LESSON FOUR

A NEW APPROACH

You've heard it all before: "Set your goals and meet them!" "You can do anything you want to and be as thin as you want to if you're willing to make the sacrifice." "Don't give up. Try harder!" "Stay away from those fattening foods. Just use a little will power!" "Lose 30 pounds in 30 days or your money back!"

Smug exhortations and carefully planned slogans have left many of us feeling like a total failure when we don't see the desired results. Many have reported to me that when a guaranteed (perhaps even fraudulent) product failed, they didn't even return it because they were sure it was *they* who had failed, not the product.

We don't use catchy slogans. We don't make ridiculous claims or outlandish guarantees. We only make one promise: If you follow this program exactly as it's outlined, you'll be changed—from the inside out.

With that promise, we take a different approach. In the next five days we'll explore five different aspects of our strategy.

Read *The All-New Free to Be Thin*—Chapters 5 and 7.

GOALS FOR THIS WEEK:

- To have a daily quiet time using the Scripture readings assigned.
- To recognize changes I need to make in
  - _____
  - _____
  - _____
- Other goals:

_____
_____
_____
_____

DAY ONE   **READ 2 CORINTHIANS 5:1–10**

A NEW GOAL

God is impressing on me that . . .

I've shared with the Lord that . . .

Thought for the Day:

I will be held accountable, not for how I look, but for what I have done.

Today's Challenge:

God is pleased with me today because:
1. I am . . .
2. I seek . . .
3. I want . . .

Food Choices	How Many?	Exchange Group:

Total Exchanges

Bread	Meat	Vegetable	Fruit	Milk	Fat

DAY TWO   **READ 1 SAMUEL 15:22**

A BETTER WAY

God is impressing on me that . . .

I've shared with the Lord that . . .

Thought for the Day:

My success is not a matter of how much I give up, but of how much I submit to God and His loving, caring will for my life.

Today's Challenge:

I will make today more a matter of obedience than sacrifice.

Food Choices	How Many?	Exchange Group:

Total Exchanges

Bread	Meat	Vegetable	Fruit	Milk	Fat

DAY THREE   READ PHILIPPIANS 2:12–14
NOT ME, BUT GOD.

God is impressing on me that . . .

I've shared with the Lord that . . .

Thought for the Day:

God is not working *on* me, but *in* me. What's the difference?

Today's Challenge:

Today I will look for God at work in me in the following ways:

Food Choices			How Many?	Exchange Group:

Total Exchanges

Bread	Meat	Vegetable	Fruit	Milk	Fat

God is impressing on me that . . .

I've shared with the Lord that . . .

Thought for the Day:

If I am to see His power at work in me, I'll need to be plugged into the right source.

Today's Challenge:

I anticipate keeping myself connected to the only real source of strength for my new life.

Food Choices	How Many?	Exchange Group:
Total Exchanges		

Bread	Meat	Vegetable	Fruit	Milk	Fat

God is impressing on me that . . .

I've shared with the Lord that . . .

Thought for the Day:

It's not my body that needs to change as much as my heart. That could take a while. God says it's okay—He's in no hurry.

Today's Challenge:

I will take each victory and each setback with equal confidence that He is working in me.

Comments:

Food Choices				How Many?	Exchange Group:

Total Exchanges

Bread	Meat	Vegetable	Fruit	Milk	Fat

A NEW APPROACH

We started our study with the words of Isaiah: "Forget the former things; do not dwell on the past. See, I am doing a new thing!" (43:18–19). That was the beginning of a totally new approach to weight and overeating management. Let's examine a little more closely five aspects of this new approach.

1. *The goal is to please God* (2 Corinthians 5:1–10). "So we make it our goal to please Him, whether we are at home in the body or away from it" (v.9).

Most weight-loss or weight-management programs focus on weight only. We focus on much more. It is our intention to please not ourselves, but our Lord. We must realize that we can please God no matter what our size, because while others are looking on the outward appearance, God is looking on the heart. While society puts pressure on us to conform to its current popular body image, God is at work helping us conform to the image of His Son, Jesus. God is pleased with our effort and our commitment to have a heart that is pure before Him.

2. *Obedience—a better way* (1 Samuel 15:22). "Does the Lord delight in burnt offerings and sacrifices as much as in obeying the voice of the LORD? To obey is better than sacrifice, and to heed is better than the fat of rams."

It's not your outward sacrifice that God is after, but obedience from your heart. Sacrifice can be empty and ritualistic, while obedience from the heart is rich and relational.

3. *It's not I but He who is working* (Philippians 2:12–14). "For it is God who works in you to will and to act according to His good purpose" (v.13).

Only when we recognize that He is at work to solve a problem we cannot solve does our obedience make sense. An attitude of obedience carries us through the tough times, helping us rise above discouragement when the results are less than what we desire. We're not responsible for the outcome—only the obedience. He's at work, and He's working *in* me, not *on* me.

4. *Not will power, but His power* (Philippians 3:20–21). "By the power that enables Him to bring everything under His control, He will transform our lowly bodies so that they will be like His glorious body" (v.21).

Yielding to His control in my life, bending and even blending into His will for my life, accomplishes what He desires for me. It's His job to accomplish—mine to obey.

5. *There's no hurry!* (Philippians 1:6). "Being confident of this, that He who began a good work in you will carry it on to completion until the day of Christ Jesus."

God is not under a deadline. He doesn't force you and pound you into losing two dress sizes before the class reunion or thirty-five pounds before your son's wedding, only to let you gain back ten before the reception is over. He's doing a work that will last a lifetime. It isn't your body He's changing—it's *you*, from the heart. Furthermore, as the Master of the Universe, He has all the time there is to do what He wants to do!

Focusing on each of these aspects of a new approach, which gives you the greatest challenge?

_____

_____

_____

Which gives you the most hope?

_____

_____

_____

How are the challenge and your hope related?

_____

_____

_____

When you review your calorie limit and your food choices of the past week in light of these five biblical principles, how does your perspective change with regard to previous attempts at weight or overeating management?

_____

_____

_____

_____

Write your response to the idea of a longer, slower approach to change and weight or overeating management:

_____

_____

_____

If you are working through this journal alone, turn to the Leader's Notes for Lesson Four on page 250 and follow the directions for the study of a passage from Haggai. Write the answers to your questions below. If you are in a study group, your group leader will give you instructions for using this space.

My first response to the passage from Haggai:

_____

_____

_____

My second response to the passage from Haggai:

_____

_____

_____

Further response to this passage after others have shared:

_____

_____

_____

WEEKLY EVALUATION

Goals for the week that I have seen realized:

_____
_____
_____

Goals that were set but only partially realized:

_____
_____
_____

Goals I will carry over to next week because they are worthwhile
and important to me:

_____
_____
_____

Goals that I will drop or adjust because they were unrealistic or
unimportant:

_____
_____

The most important thing I learned from this week's lesson:

_____
_____
_____

A victory I would like to record:

_____
_____
_____

I am surrendering to God . . .

_____
_____
_____

I am choosing to be more obedient to God in . . .

_____
_____
_____

A NEW FOCUS

It's an unusual weight-management program that encourages you to stay away from the scale, wouldn't you agree? But our approach does just that, and for good reason.

Think of how you feel when you step on the scale. We've trained ourselves to believe that if the reading is lower than it was the time before, then the *program* is working. If the scale reports no change in weight, we raise our eyebrows and determine to do better—usually meaning we'll eat less. If the scale reports a gain—*oh, no!*—we usually feel like a failure and begin our search for another program or plan.

It's almost time to weigh again, but with an entirely new focus. The next five readings will help you put that focus into place.

▶ Read *The All-New Free to Be Thin*—Chapter 6.

Goals for This Week:

- To have a daily quiet time using the Scripture readings assigned.
- To recognize changes I need to make in
    - _____
    - _____
    - _____
- Other goals:

_____
_____
_____
_____

God is impressing on me that . . .

I've shared with the Lord that . . .

Thought for the Day:

What lies behind, or even all around, is not as important as what lies ahead.

Today's Challenge:

Today I will look ahead with confidence.

Food Choices	How Many?	Exchange Group:

Total Exchanges

Bread	Meat	Vegetable	Fruit	Milk	Fat

God is impressing on me that . . .

I've shared with the Lord that . . .

Thought for the Day:

Essential to our success is looking at what God is doing, not at what I *think* He should be doing.

Today's Challenge:

I determine to discover and acknowledge what God is doing in me.

Food Choices	How Many?	Exchange Group:

Total Exchanges					
Bread	Meat	Vegetable	Fruit	Milk	Fat

God is impressing on me that . . .

I've shared with the Lord that . . .

Thought for the Day:

Jesus knows what pain is. Let Him be your comfort and strength today.

Today's Challenge:

I plan to "fix my mind" on Jesus today.

Food Choices	How Many?	Exchange Group:

Total Exchanges

Bread	Meat	Vegetable	Fruit	Milk	Fat

LOOKING TO GOD

God is impressing on me that . . .

I've shared with the Lord that . . .

Thought for the Day:

The scale only says how much you *weigh*—not how much you're *worth*. What's the difference?

Today's Challenge:

I will see my worth in God based on His love for me. (See John 3:16.)

Food Choices			How Many?	Exchange Group:

Total Exchanges					
Bread	Meat	Vegetable	Fruit	Milk	Fat

DAY FIVE **READ 2 CHRONICLES 16:9**
GOD IS LOOKING AT YOU!

God is impressing on me that . . .

I've shared with the Lord that . . .

Thought for the Day:

God is looking at you and He likes what He sees!

Comments:

Today's Challenge:

I resolve to submit to God based on my commitment to Him.

Food Choices	How Many?	Exchange Group:

Total Exchanges

Bread	Meat	Vegetable	Fruit	Milk	Fat

LESSON FIVE

A NEW FOCUS

It's so easy to focus on the program, our progress, or even the process and miss the miracle of God's involvement in our lives. As strange as it seems, this is why we encourage you to weigh only three times during this study. You see, changing weight doesn't change you! Only the Lord can change you, and if you find the scale not cooperating, you may begin to believe that He's not working. The old mindset that the program isn't working will only be transferred to our relationship with God.

Stay off the scale? No, not entirely, but weigh for a reason that's different from before. This time when you weigh, your focus will be not on weight loss, but on five essential biblical insights.

INSIGHT NUMBER ONE

Focus: Looking ahead. "Let your eyes look straight ahead, fix your gaze directly before you" (Proverbs 4:25).

It's so easy to look back—back over a disastrous week or back at a former weight-loss method that worked, even though it was followed by regain. But that habit can be counterproductive to the work God is doing in you now. We have a past, of course, but we live in the present. We learn from the past, yes, but we must look toward the future.

INSIGHT NUMBER TWO

Focus: Looking above. "Since, then, you have been raised with Christ, set your hearts on things above, where Christ is seated at the right hand of God. Set your minds on things above, not on earthly things" (Colossians 3:1-2).

It's so easy to look around. Most weight groups announce the weight-loss winners each week. Only one person can lose the most weight, but in OV we believe that God is working in every one of us. We recognize that weight loss varies from person to person, and that the person losing the most weight is not necessarily the winner with regard to seeing God at work in his or her life. Looking above keeps our focus off ourselves and on what God is doing.

INSIGHT NUMBER THREE

Focus: Looking to Jesus. "Let us fix our eyes on Jesus, the author and perfecter of our faith, who for the joy set before Him endured the cross, scorning its shame, and sat down at the right hand of the throne of God. Consider Him who endured such opposition from sinful men, so that you will not grow weary and lose heart" (Hebrews 12:2–3).

It sometimes gets worse before it gets better. No one knows that better than Jesus. He can give you the most understanding when it gets tough. He went through what He did with a purpose in mind, and that purpose was *you*. You were His focus then; let Him be yours now.

INSIGHT NUMBER FOUR

Focus: Looking to God. "Those who look to Him are radiant; their faces are never covered with shame" (Psalm 34:5).

No matter what the scale says, your face will be radiant if you're looking to God. He is at work in you. The scale only tells you how much you weigh, not how much you're worth.

INSIGHT NUMBER FIVE

Focus: God is looking at me! "For the eyes of the Lord range throughout the earth to strengthen those whose hearts are fully committed to him" (2 Chronicles 16:9).

Picture this: You're standing on the scale looking at the dial while God is in heaven watching for your commitment, your total submission to Him and your recognition of what He's doing in your life. He gives you the strength to weigh for the right reason. Remember your victory was bought on the cross—not on the scale.

Then what's the right reason to weigh? Not to encourage

you—that's what the Word of God, this study, and your group are for. (Of course, if a weight loss is registered, you *will* be encouraged.) Not to scold you or to make you feel like a failure. The scale can't measure your obedience or commitment. It can only measure your bodily weight.

The reason for weighing is that right about now, you *need* to know how much you weigh so you can re-compute your calorie needs and make the adjustments necessary in your daily food selections. So as you weigh, keep the right focus.

Before you go to your class, if you are in a group study, take some time to think about the following "what if's." Write your responses in the space provided.

What if the scale shows you're losing weight?

How will that affect you emotionally?

_____

_____

How will that affect your commitment to complete this study?

_____

_____

How will that affect your faith?

_____

_____

How will that affect your food choices?

_____

_____

What if the scale shows you've stayed the same weight?

How will that affect you emotionally?

_____

_____

How will that affect your commitment to complete this study?

_____

_____

How will that affect your faith?

_____

_____

How will that affect your food choices?

_____

_____

What if the scale shows you have gained some weight since the beginning of this study?

How will that affect you emotionally?

_____

How will that affect your commitment to complete this study?

_____

How will that affect your faith?

_____

How will that affect your food choices?

_____

How can you prepare yourself to weigh?

_____

Would you rather weigh at your group or by yourself? Why?

_____

Whether you weigh at your group of by yourself, record your weight:

Weight: _____   Change: _____

                                       Loss (−)

                                       Same (0)

                                       Gain (+)

How did your preparation help you accept the scale reading?

_____

How are you adjusting your calorie limit?

_____

Weekly Evaluation

Goals for the week that I have seen realized:

_____
_____
_____

Goals that were set but only partially realized:

_____
_____
_____

Goals I will carry over to next week because they are worthwhile
and important to me:

_____
_____
_____

Goals that I will drop or adjust because they were unrealistic or
unimportant:

_____
_____

The most important thing I learned from this week's lesson:

_____
_____
_____

A victory I would like to record:

_____
_____
_____

I am surrendering to God . . .

_____
_____
_____

I am choosing to be more obedient to God in . . .

_____
_____
_____

A Renewed Commitment

This is your moment! The step you take in this lesson is even more crucial to your success at being free than the one you took to begin this study.

You have an important decision to make: to give up or to go on. It's up to you.

The time immediately following a weight-check is when many Free-to-Be-Thinners find themselves at a crossroads. Make this the turning point in your life. Say "yes" to victory and put your faith to work!

Do it by making up your mind to renew your commitment to change. The following five quiet times are designed to help you:

1. Choose to walk in obedience.
2. Choose to walk in the Spirit.
3. Make up your mind to live more for Christ than for self.
4. Find your delight in the Lord and in Him alone.
5. Learn to wait on the Lord.

Read *The All-New Free to Be Thin*—Chapters 15–17, 20.

Goals for This Week

- To have a daily quiet time using the Scripture readings assigned.
- To recognize changes I need to make in
    - _____
    - _____
    - _____
- Other goals:

_____
_____
_____
_____

God is impressing on me that . . .

I've shared with the Lord that . . .

Thought for the Day:

I've been chosen for obedience.
Comments:

Today's Challenge:

I will remain aware of being chosen for obedience today by . . .

Food Choices	How Many?	Exchange Group:

Total Exchanges

Bread	Meat	Vegetable	Fruit	Milk	Fat

God is impressing on me that . . .

I've shared with the Lord that . . .

Thought for the Day:

The Spirit-controlled mind is not an issue of possession, but submission.

Today's Challenge:

I determine practice focusing on the Holy Spirit.

Food Choices	How Many?	Exchange Group:

Total Exchanges

Bread	Meat	Vegetable	Fruit	Milk	Fat

DAY THREE   **READ 2 CORINTHIANS 5:14–15**
LIVING FOR CHRIST

God is impressing on me that . . .

I've shared with the Lord that . . .

Thought for the Day:

If I lived more for Christ and less for myself, how would that change how I deal with anger, temptation, and impatience with other people?

Today's Challenge:

I choose to consciously live more for Christ than for myself today.

Food Choices	How Many?	Exchange Group:

Total Exchanges

Bread	Meat	Vegetable	Fruit	Milk	Fat

God is impressing on me that . . .

I've shared with the Lord that . . .

Thought for the Day:

Intimacy with the Lord will only come when we take the time and make the effort to be with Him.

Today's Challenge:

I will gaze upon the beauty of the Lord and to delight in Him.

Food Choices	How Many?	Exchange Group:

Total Exchanges

Bread	Meat	Vegetable	Fruit	Milk	Fat

DAY FIVE   **READ ISAIAH 30:18-20**

WAITING ON GOD

God is impressing on me that . . .

I've shared with the Lord that . . .

Thought for the Day:

Because the Lord knows what He's doing and can see the final result, He's in no hurry!
Comments:

Today's Challenge:

I choose to wait on God today.

Food Choices	How Many?	Exchange Group:

Total Exchanges

Bread	Meat	Vegetable	Fruit	Milk	Fat

A RENEWED COMMITMENT

Chosen to chose obedience, what an awesome thought! I was not chosen because I am a particularly good choice. I'm not the best-looking, most talented, or even the most likely to succeed. But God sees potential in me. He sees the potential that I can *obey*. I have not been chosen to produce results, but through obedience reproduce His likeness. I cannot see the results in a mirror, but only reflected in His face. I cannot measure the results with a tape measure, but only as I conform to His Word and see the changes in my life.

It is essential that I learn that my success is directly in proportion to God's Holy Spirit's power living in and through me. I cannot manipulate God to work in me, nor can I manipulate any lasting success by *zapping* my problem areas with His Word as though it were an electric cattle prod. No, it is only as I choose to obey and allow Him to live in me that I discover His power working through me.

Living for Christ changes everything. It changes my attitudes toward other people, attitudes toward my work and my church. It changes how I pick friends, and how often I read my Bible. Living for Christ even changes how I make food choices.

However, living for Christ does not happen apart from my conscious moment-by-moment decision. Just as the butterfly doesn't wake up one morning and spread its colorful wings free of the cocoon, I, too, often find myself fighting my way to freedom. But the struggle is not for freedom—that is my destiny—my struggle is what produces the strength to fly once I am free.

Delighting in the Lord requires that we make room in our hearts for Him. But it also requires room in our busy schedules. Intimacy with Christ cannot happen without private time with Him. That is what this study has been giving you. Once you finish this thirteen-week series, you may walk away from this book never to pick it up again, but I guarantee this: You will never be able to live without intimacy with Christ and be satisfied again.

Once we begin to live more for Him than for ourselves, once we discover delightful intimacy with Him—then it becomes easier to wait on Him. We can rest in assurance that He is working in our hearts and lives, and that He has a special purpose for each of us. He can see the final results we can only hope for.

It's time to make your choice. Are you giving up or going on? Are you deciding to turn back or are you choosing to let God work a change in you no matter what you weigh?

It's an important decision to make, and no one can make it for you. It's totally up to you. The time for renewed commitment is now!

Write out words to express your inner feelings: _____

_____

_____

Write out your fears concerning totally surrendering your weight management to God: _____

_____

_____

If a person does not surrender this effort to Him, can they say that they have a totally surrendered their life to God's will?

_____

_____

What is your decision? Are you going back, or going on? _____

_____

_____

Explain your decision to God in writing: _____

_____

_____

_____

_____

WEEKLY EVALUATION

Goals for the week that I have seen realized:
_____
_____
_____

Goals that were set but only partially realized:
_____
_____
_____

Goals I will carry over to next week because they are worthwhile and important to me:
_____
_____
_____

Goals that I will drop or adjust because they were unrealistic or unimportant:
_____
_____

The most important thing I learned from this week's lesson:
_____
_____
_____

A victory I would like to record:
_____
_____
_____

I am surrendering to God . . .
_____
_____
_____

I am choosing to be more obedient to God in . . .
_____
_____
_____

PREPARATION FOR LESSON SEVEN

A NEW LIFESTYLE

In previous weeks of this study, we've been adding new concepts to new habits for one reason: to build a new lifestyle, the All-New Free to Be Thin Lifestyle.

This week, in addition to the five quiet times, food selections, and evening reflections, we add one more crucial lifestyle change—physical exercise.

I've deliberately avoided using Scripture texts about discipline or training the body for good reason: We have come to embrace this new lifestyle, not as a matter of *should's*, but as a matter of responsible *choices*.

It's important that we take responsibility for our physical bodies, not because we *have* to, but because we *choose* to do for our bodies whatever we know to be healthy and wise.

This week I encourage you to explore, even experiment with, several exercise options—walking, personal exercise video tapes, or a low-impact aerobics class. You can find a walking program, "Step by Step," described in Appendix G. If you prefer an exercise video, I recommend either Stormie Omartian's *First Step* or Overeater Victorious's own *Fit for a King* with Stormie and myself, along with five other Free-to-Be-Thinners (Sparrow).

Now, as you incorporate physical exercise, enjoy your new lifestyle.

📖 Read *The All-New Free to Be Thin*—Chapters 8–11

GOALS FOR THIS WEEK

- To have a daily quiet time using the Scripture readings assigned.
- To recognize changes I need to make in
  - _____
  - _____
  - _____
- Exercise goal (choose one):
  - ☐ walking _____ minutes per day.
  - ☐ low-impact aerobics class _____ times this week
  - ☐ low-impact aerobics video tape(title) _____ times this week.
- Other goals:

_____
_____
_____
_____

DAY ONE   **READ PSALM 32:1-7**

HONESTY WITH GOD

God is impressing on me that . . .

I've shared with the Lord that . . .

Thought for the Day:

My way is not kept blameless through tremendous effort toward perfection, but through honesty and openness, confessing my shortcomings as soon as I discover them.

Today's Challenge:

In honesty and openness I stand before God with the following personal issues:

Food Choices	How Many?	Exchange Group:
Total Exchanges		

Bread	Meat	Vegetable	Fruit	Milk	Fat

God is impressing on me that . . .

I've shared with the Lord that . . .

Thought for the Day:

Through daily Bible reading, I am able to tuck God's Word deep into the secret places of my heart, places where I might otherwise tuck the secrets of self.

Today's Challenge:

Areas of my heart I will open to God and His Word:

Food Choices	How Many?	Exchange Group:

Total Exchanges

Bread	Meat	Vegetable	Fruit	Milk	Fat

God is impressing on me that . . .

I've shared with the Lord that . . .

Thought for the Day:

Help me to see, Lord, that I owe a debt of gratitude to anything that causes me to turn to You.

Today's Challenge:

I will turn to the Lord today with or without special motivation.

Food Choices	How Many?	Exchange Group:

Total Exchanges

Bread	Meat	Vegetable	Fruit	Milk	Fat

God is impressing on me that . . .

I've shared with the Lord that . . .

Thought for the Day:

When I consider my ways, the mistakes I've made, the pain I've felt and even caused myself, I say, "Lord, Your way is better."

Today's Challenge:

Today I will choose God's way over my own by . . .

Food Choices				How Many?	Exchange Group:

Total Exchanges

Bread	Meat	Vegetable	Fruit	Milk	Fat

WEEK SEVEN	DAY FIVE	READ GALATIANS 3:23-25
		A NEW FREEDOM

God is impressing on me that . . .

I've shared with the Lord that . . .

Thought for the Day:

God is not interested in penning us up, but in setting us free.

Today's Challenge:

Today I will walk in new freedom by . . .

Food Choices	How Many?	Exchange Group:

Total Exchanges

Bread	Meat	Vegetable	Fruit	Milk	Fat

LESSON SEVEN

A New Lifestyle

Not a new body—a new lifestyle. A lifestyle free of shame. A lifestyle with no disgrace or embarrassment or guilt. Free-to-Be-Thinners live a life of balanced control, and experience the freedom and joy of responsible choice. Obsessions and extremes are left far behind along with self-hatred and other destructive attitudes and habits.

Fad diets with their daily promises no longer deceive us. TV commercials with empty claims no longer hold the allure they once did. Scales no longer dictate our destinies or define our worth.

This is a completely new approach, and we love it for good reason. Our new lifestyle is based on God's Word, experienced in daily loving relationship with Him. The changes taking place are coming from the inside out.

Our new way of life is based on the privilege of delighting in God's law, rejoicing in His Word, and gaining a new understanding of ourselves and the dynamics of our relationship with our heavenly Father. With Him as our source, we discover new determination and unlimited strength to choose the new freedom He offers.

The strength of this lifestyle enables Free-to-Be-Thinners to eat what's good and to identify and refuse what's best left alone. It motivates us to become more physically active because exercise is a healthy, lovely discipline. It encourages us to evaluate our worth in light of God's love, to bless our bodies, souls, and spirits by making good choices and healthy decisions. It energizes us to keep our commitments, gives us the compassion to forgive ourselves, and empowers us to recover when we stumble.

In light of the wonderful insights you've learned since you've adopted the All-New Free to Be Thin Lifestyle for yourself, answer the following questions:

1. Someone has defined God's law as "the whole of God's revealed will." With that definition in mind, why do you think some of us still separate God's law from His love?

_____

_____

_____

2. Drawing from your own experience, what does it mean to you to see God's law (His known will) and His love as inseparable?

_____

_____

_____

3. What happens when we separate God's love from His law?

_____

_____

4. What inner changes result from rejoicing in God's Word?

_____

_____

_____

5. What new insights do you now have in
   Food choices:

_____

_____

_____

   Weight management:

_____

_____

_____

   Physical exercise:

_____

_____

_____

   Other new insights since beginning this program:

_____

_____

_____

_____

6. How has your determination to change been strengthened since starting this study?

_____

_____

_____

_____

7. What freedom do you now have that you didn't before?

_____

_____

_____

8. What form of exercise have you decided to try?

_____

Weekly Evaluation

Goals for the week that I have seen realized:
_____
_____
_____

Goals that were set but only partially realized:
_____
_____
_____

Goals I will carry over to next week because they are worthwhile
and important to me:
_____
_____
_____

Goals that I will drop or adjust because they were unrealistic or
unimportant:
_____
_____

The most important thing I learned from this week's lesson:
_____
_____
_____

A victory I would like to record:
_____
_____
_____

I am surrendering to God . . .
_____
_____
_____

I am choosing to be more obedient to God in . . .
_____
_____
_____

A NEW THING

I know it may be hard to believe, but the best just got better! As if a new focus and a new approach weren't enough, God gives us a new lifestyle. Then, before we can fully begin to understand just how much He's done, He keeps on giving. This time, He gives us what the prophet Isaiah calls "a new thing" (Isaiah 43:19)—some gift of grace added on top of everything else that surprises and amazes us.

The next five daily quiet times will enrich your life and help you see the fresh new thing God is doing in your heart and life, whatever it may be. Perhaps it's a new zest for life or a new depth in your marriage relationship. God is sure to surprise you with an unexpected blessing of one sort or another.

Take the promises personally. Read them slowly; enjoy them fully. Meditate on them during your exercise program and repeat them to yourself while preparing dinner or packing your lunch for work.

God's promises are the key to your success. His Word awakens your spirit and opens the way to a life of control. My prayer is that this lesson will bring such freshness and newness that you'll gain a whole new perspective on the new thing God is about to surprise you with in your life.

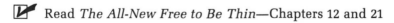 Read *The All-New Free to Be Thin*—Chapters 12 and 21

GOALS FOR THIS WEEK

- To have a daily quiet time using the Scripture readings assigned.
- To recognize changes I need to make in
    - _____
    - _____
    - _____
- Exercise goal (choose one):
    - ☐ walking _____ minutes per day.
    - ☐ low-impact aerobics class _____ times this week
    - ☐ low-impact aerobics video tape(title) _____ times this week.

_____
_____
_____

- Other goals:

_____
_____
_____
_____

God is impressing on me that . . .

I've shared with the Lord that . . .

Thought for the Day:

The new covenant is not based on what we have done, but on who God is.

Today's Challenge:

I will base today's success on who God is.

Food Choices	How Many?	Exchange Group:

Total Exchanges

Bread	Meat	Vegetable	Fruit	Milk	Fat

DAY TWO **READ 1 CORINTHIANS 9:25**

NEW PURPOSE

God is impressing on me that . . .

I've shared with the Lord that . . .

Thought for the Day:

You cannot run to win without first training to run.
Comments:

Today's Challenge:

I choose to submit myself to God's training.

Food Choices	How Many?	Exchange Group:

Total Exchanges

Bread	Meat	Vegetable	Fruit	Milk	Fat

God is impressing on me that . . .

I've shared with the Lord that . . .

Thought for the Day:

If my body is not to be my master, it must become my slave.

Comments:

Today's Challenge:

I determine to be in control of my eating habits with God's help.

Food Choices	How Many?	Exchange Group:

Total Exchanges

Bread	Meat	Vegetable	Fruit	Milk	Fat

DAY FOUR   **READ COLOSSIANS 1:9–10**
                    NEW UNDERSTANDING

God is impressing on me that . . .

I've shared with the Lord that . . .

Thought for the Day:

We don't measure success by pounds and inches lost, but by gaining in the knowledge of God.
Comments:

Today's Challenge:

I expect to know God better through each trial or victory.

Food Choices	How Many?	Exchange Group:

Total Exchanges

Bread	Meat	Vegetable	Fruit	Milk	Fat

DAY FIVE

READ COLOSSIANS 1:11-12

NEW POWER

God is impressing on me that . . .

I've shared with the Lord that . . .

Thought for the Day:

Our success is not dependent on our ability to say no to temptation, but on our decision to say yes to God.
Comments:

Today's Challenge:

The new thing God is doing in me will help me to face temptation differently. For example . . .

Food Choices	How Many?	Exchange Group:

Total Exchanges

Bread	Meat	Vegetable	Fruit	Milk	Fat

A NEW THING

These lessons have offered you a novel approach to weight and overeating management, don't you agree? For many, this exciting new way to approach these two difficult issues has been a radical departure from the old ways that we've tried to become thin and acceptable.

But becoming thin can never be the basis for acceptability to God. No, God doesn't like thin people more than He likes you! I've met many thin people who were once large, and now that they've arrived at thin, they're in even more bondage than when they were fat. That won't happen to you if you join us in focusing on the freedom and the exciting new thing God is doing within you that will sustain you, thin or not!

First, God promises a new covenant. His people includes you if you have accepted His Son Jesus as your personal Savior. Simply inviting Christ into your life qualifies you for every promise of the Bible.

Hidden deep within certain prophecies are promises for God's children as they reveal the heart of the Father. Consider these in Jeremiah 31:31–37:

1. God will not pull us along by the hand, but instead He will write His law on our hearts and give us the choice to obey them.

2. He promises to be our God and to make us His people.

3. Our past sins have been reckoned with. God has taken care of them and will not hold our past against us any longer.

4. We will forever be His children. Forever!

5. We will *never* be rejected by Him for anything we've ever done!

God's covenant is not based on our performance, but on His.

That's the best deal in town, wouldn't you agree? Imagine getting an offer in which everything I've ever done, all the ways I've been disqualified as the recipient, have been done away with. All I'm required to do is accept the offer.

No wonder we feel a great sense of renewed purpose welling up within us. No wonder we sense a great love springing up in our hearts, wanting to burst forth in praise and adoration to our God. No wonder we begin to train our physical bodies out of gratitude and a new sense of responsibility and purpose.

In this new approach we probe our inner hearts and uncover the excuses we have used for so many years to stay in bondage to food and inactivity. We begin to embrace scriptural passages that encourage us to take better care of our bodies, responding with a resounding "Yes"!

In our new covenant relationship with God, we gain a new understanding that success is found in knowing Him and that the process we're now going through is giving us the opportunity to experience that in a new way. We face every hurdle knowing our power to resist is not found in saying no to temptation but in saying yes to God.

In Overeaters Victorious we've changed the rules. We've made great strides in understanding the overweight or overeating Christian. We won't settle for the same old worldly attitudes about body image, and succumb to societal pressure to conform to a certain dress size any longer. We choose instead a life of controlled, healthful choices. We choose to exercise our bodies out of gratitude to God for them, whatever their size. We choose to love ourselves with a healthy God-inspired love, and to choose good food that blesses rather than curses our bodies.

As we make all these new choices, God is at work blessing us with freshness and renewal in every area of our lives. Often the "new thing" He does will go beyond our expectations and even surprise us. The apostle Paul said it best: God "is able to do immeasurably more than all we ask or imagine, according to His power that is at work within us" (Ephesians 3:20).

Answer the following questions:

1. Can you express in your own words the surprising new thing that you sense God doing in you that doesn't seem to be related to your weight or eating habits?

_____

_____

_____

_____

_____

_____

2. What new and surprising thing do you sense God doing in you that *is* related to your weight or eating habits?

_____

_____

_____

3. What new thing has happened to you concerning exercise?

_____

_____

_____

4. What new feelings do you have about yourself?

_____

_____

_____

_____

WEEKLY EVALUATION

Goals for the week that I have seen realized:
_____
_____
_____

Goals that were set but only partially realized:
_____
_____
_____

Goals I will carry over to next week because they are worthwhile
and important to me:
_____
_____
_____

Goals that I will drop or adjust because they were unrealistic or
unimportant:
_____
_____

The most important thing I learned from this week's lesson:
_____
_____
_____

A victory I would like to record:
_____
_____
_____

I am surrendering to God . . .
_____
_____
_____

I am choosing to be more obedient to God in . . .
_____
_____
_____

THE NEW YOU

If you're like most people, you probably expect to see in the bathroom mirror the evidence of being a brand-new person. Yet you probably also have noticed that the changes reflected in the mirror can be so small they're almost overlooked. Nevertheless, the changes on the inside, the ones that are hidden, are tremendous—almost miraculous.

Our society insists that if you're in a weight-management course, you should be dropping pounds and inches every day. But that's not necessarily true. Worse yet, some well-meaning but misinformed Christians also believe that as you bring the body into line with culturally accepted norms, Jesus will love you more and be more pleased with you. Nothing could be further from the truth.

This is not a self-improvement course; it's a personal-growth course. Growing in the knowledge of our Lord and Savior Jesus Christ will have an impact on your physical body, but losing weight in itself won't bring you closer to God. Jesus couldn't be happier with you or love you any more than He does right now.

It's not a new body He's giving—it's a new you. A *whole* new you. This week's Scripture readings will focus on that new person you're becoming. Let God's Word be the mirror of the real and eternal work He's doing.

Read *The All-New Free to Be Thin*—Chapters 13–14

Goals for This Week:

- To have a daily quiet time using the Scripture readings assigned.
- To recognize changes I need to make in
  - _____
  - _____
  - _____
- Exercise goal (choose one):
  - ☐ walking _____ minutes per day.
  - ☐ low-impact aerobics class _____ times this week.
  - ☐ low-impact aerobics video tape(title) _____ times this week.

_____

_____

_____

- Other goals:

_____

_____

_____

_____

DAY ONE   **READ EPHESIANS 1:3-8**
SONS AND DAUGHTERS OF GOD

God is impressing on me that . . .

I've shared with the Lord that . . .

Thought for the Day:

In Christ my life is not as much about making new changes and choices as it is about becoming a new person. Comments:

Today's Challenge:

In Christ I am a new person, and I will show it in the following ways:

Food Choices				How Many?	Exchange Group:

Total Exchanges

Bread	Meat	Vegetable	Fruit	Milk	Fat

DAY TWO READ EPHESIANS 1:9–14; 1 PETER 1:3–5
MY FULL INHERITANCE

God is impressing on me that . . .

I've shared with the Lord that . . .

Thought for the Day:

While I can't physically see or touch Jesus, I can by faith let Jesus touch me. Comments:

Today's Challenge:

Knowing I have a full inheritance waiting for me will change how I approach my struggles today in the following ways:

Food Choices				How Many?	Exchange Group:

Total Exchanges

Bread	Meat	Vegetable	Fruit	Milk	Fat

God is impressing on me that . . .

I've shared with the Lord that . . .

Thought for the day:

Experiencing Christ's righteousness, holiness, and redemption not only changes how I see Him but how I see myself!

Comments:

Today's Challenge:

Today I will walk in my new identity. I anticipate a difference in the following ways:

Food Choices	How Many?	Exchange Group:

Total Exchanges

Bread	Meat	Vegetable	Fruit	Milk	Fat

God is impressing on me that . . .

I've shared with the Lord that . . .

Thought for the day:

The God who chooses us, adopts us, gives freely to us, even lavishes gifts upon us, also disciplines us lest we become spoiled children.

Today's Challenge:

I will see God's loving hand of discipline today in the following ways:

Food Choices				How Many?	Exchange Group:

Total Exchanges

Bread	Meat	Vegetable	Fruit	Milk	Fat

God is impressing on me that . . .

I've shared with the Lord that . . .

Thought for the Day:

Focusing on our position in Christ helps us live above
our struggles—not under them.
Comments:

Today's Challenge:

Today, because of my position in Christ, I will rise
above my struggles:

Food Choices				How Many?	Exchange Group:
Total Exchanges					
Bread	Meat	Vegetable	Fruit	Milk	Fat

THE NEW YOU

Did you know that according to Scripture we have everything we need for a truly victorious life? God's power has provided us with all we need for life and godliness (2 Peter 1:3). We have justification, sanctification, and perfection (1 Corinthians 1:30). We also have every spiritual blessing in the heavenly places in Christ (Ephesians 1:3).

In Jesus we have been seated in the heavenlies with God (Ephesians 2:6). How is it then, you may ask, that we sometimes don't experience this heavenly life moment by moment? If I am a new me, why do I feel much of the time like the same old frumpy failure?

As Christians we know we're to "grow up" in Christ. We're to be constantly maturing. So we may become discouraged when we focus on our day-to-day progress with its momentary struggles and perhaps defeats. That's why it's best to focus on our identity in Christ rather than on our progress.

If we were to graph our progress, we'd see that the lessons learned from each struggle and failure can—if we let them have their full work within us—bring us ever closer to the fullness of our *position* in Christ. We can actually benefit from our failure. Of course, we can't use this insight as an excuse to fail. But when we *do* fail, we can view the situation as only a momentary slip from which we can gain experience and growth.

God has planned a way to bring us out of struggles into victory, to move us closer to Jesus, and to make us more the overcomers He promised we would be. His way is *repentance*—a simple process of confessing our wrongdoing and turning away from it to go on with Him; a constant yielding and surrendering to God. The Holy Spirit enables us to walk more and more victoriously as we daily yield to Him.

Our union with Christ and our daily struggles can be represented on a chart this way:

"WE ARE SEATED WITH CHRIST IN THE HEAVENLIES"
(Eph. 1:3; 2:6)
Positional justification, sanctification, perfection
(1 Cor. 1:30)

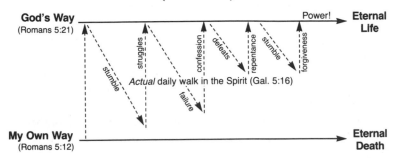

When we reckon ourselves dead to sin and alive to God through the cross of Christ (see Romans 6:11), and we die daily (see 1 Corinthians 15:31), the Holy Spirit enables us to have victory over sin and self, over old habits of thinking, doing, and reacting. Keeping in clear focus our position in Christ while living out the day-by-day experiences helps us to overcome, to become victorious, and to walk in power.

You are secure in Jesus. Your day-to-day struggles don't change your position—your identity—in Christ. Even though many times you may feel as if you've lost your position in Christ, your identity in Him actually remains the same.

Since you've accepted Jesus as your Savior, you are a son or daughter to Christ, no matter what! (See Ephesians 1:3–8.) Even if you totally desert Him and turn your back on Him, the moment you *return* to Him, He'll be found waiting for you. No matter how many times you blow your eating plan or sabotage your prayerfully established goals, when you open yourself to the loving, waiting Savior you'll find your inheritance as His child still deposited in your account—held in trust for you (see Ephesians 1:9; 1 Peter 1:3–4).

Even though you may have been trained throughout your entire life to see yourself as a failure and of no value, in Jesus you have a new identity (see 1 Corinthians 1:26–31). In Christ you are a victor, an overcomer, and a perseverer!

Though you may have always claimed to be an undisciplined person, in Christ you have become a person of discipline (see Hebrews 12:5–10)—a fact so important that we'll concentrate more on it in a later chapter.

Every insecurity you've ever experienced must give way to the security available to you in Christ. You are His; He is yours. That security has nothing to do with body size, body image, or your perfect adherence to a prescribed program of behavioral change. It has nothing to do with *your* performance, but with His (see Ephesians 1:3; 2:6).

Can you look at Scripture and focus more on your position in Jesus than on your struggles? If you can, then I guarantee you'll gain the proper perspective on your struggles, and you'll experience hope instead of despair as you move out of defeat into victory.

The new you may not show in the mirror or on the bathroom scale—*yet*. But it will show in a thousand other ways that reflect your new identity in Christ.

Answer the following questions:

When do you feel the best about your reflection in the mirror?

_____

_____

When do you best grow spiritually: When everything is going smoothly, or when there are things to overcome?

_____

Explain.

_____

_____

How does the following verse underscore this lesson?
"If we confess our sins, He is faithful and just and will forgive us our sins and purify us from all unrighteousness" (1 John 1:9).

_____

_____

What are the dangers of realizing that our position is more important than our progress?

_____

_____

How can you avoid these dangers?

_____

_____

How have you changed since beginning this study?

_____

_____

_____

How would you define "the new you" as you see God working
in your life?

_____

_____

_____

_____

Weekly Evaluation

Goals for the week that I have seen realized:

_____

_____

_____

Goals that were set but only partially realized:

_____

_____

_____

Goals I will carry over to next week because they are worthwhile
and important to me:

_____

_____

_____

Goals that I will drop or adjust because they were unrealistic or
unimportant:

_____

_____

The most important thing I learned from this week's lesson:

_____

_____

_____

A victory I would like to record:

_____

_____

_____

I am surrendering to God . . .

_____

_____

_____

I am choosing to be more obedient to God in . . .

_____

_____

_____

DISCIPLINE

How many times have you said to yourself, I know this is true, I know God loves me and that He's helping me, yet . . .

Don't you wish you could simply snap your fingers and have everything necessary to live the totally victorious Christian life that God offers? You have all the power of heaven and earth at your fingertips because God is working in you. Nevertheless, to apply that power, you still need to learn some basic skills—such as discipline, overcoming temptation, and perseverance. We'll spend the next three weeks looking at these particular skills one at a time—characteristics that must be developed in us through practice.

☑ Read *The All-New Free to Be Thin*—Chapter 22.

GOALS FOR THIS WEEK:

- To have a daily quiet time using the Scripture readings assigned.
- To recognize changes I need to make in
  - _____
  - _____
  - _____
- Exercise goal (choose one):
  ☐ walking _____ minutes per day.
  ☐ low-impact aerobics class _____ times this week.
  ☐ low-impact aerobics video tape(title) _____ times this week.

_____
_____
_____

- Other goals:

_____
_____
_____
_____

God is impressing on me that . . .

I've shared with the Lord that . . .

Thought for the Day:

Even the most difficult discipline speaks of God's love.

Today's Challenge:

I anticipate seeing God's loving hand extended toward me today in the midst of difficulty.

Food Choices				How Many?	Exchange Group:

Total Exchanges					
Bread	Meat	Vegetable	Fruit	Milk	Fat

DAY TWO   **READ EPHESIANS 6:10**

HIS STRENGTH IN ME

God is impressing on me that . . .

I've shared with the Lord that . . .

Thought for the Day:

Disciplined people have learned the art of getting up, dusting themselves off, and starting over.

Today's Challenge:

Today I will pick myself up if I fall down and begin again.

Food Choices			How Many?	Exchange Group:

Total Exchanges

Bread	Meat	Vegetable	Fruit	Milk	Fat

God is impressing on me that . . .

I've shared with the Lord that . . .

Thought for the Day:

As you grow in godliness, don't forget to love. Someone near you may need a hug more than an insight.

Today's Challenge:

I choose to listen to others and be open for improvement.

Food Choices	How Many?	Exchange Group:

Total Exchanges					
Bread	Meat	Vegetable	Fruit	Milk	Fat

DAY FOUR   **READ PHILIPPIANS 4:7-8**
NEW CHOICES

God is impressing on me that . . .

I've shared with the Lord that . . .

Thought for the Day:

In our troubled world—with its immoral societies, un-stable economics, political and religious scandals, and general decay—isn't it good to have Jesus?

Today's Challenge:

In all I face today I will be thankful that Jesus is with me.

Food Choices	How Many?	Exchange Group:

Total Exchanges

Bread	Meat	Vegetable	Fruit	Milk	Fat

DAY FIVE   **READ 1 CORINTHIANS 9:24-27**
NEW HABITS

God is impressing on me that . . .

I've shared with the Lord that . . .

Thought for the Day:

To insist on keeping pet sins and undisciplined habits is like running a race in scuba gear.

Today's Challenge:

Today I will train myself to . . .

Food Choices	How Many?	Exchange Group:
Total Exchanges		

Bread	Meat	Vegetable	Fruit	Milk	Fat

DISCIPLINE

Are you tired of trying to do what you know to do yet finding you can't? Are you weary with wasted effort and futile expenditure of personal emotional energy? Wouldn't you like to settle the discipline issue once and for all?

The problem is this: Discipline isn't an issue; it's a skill. And skills aren't settled; they're learned and then applied again and again.

Won't this struggle ever be over? As long as we're human beings coping with the "flesh," the struggle will continue. In the meantime, developing the skill of discipline isn't always much fun. Even the Bible says so:

"No discipline seems pleasant at the time, but painful. Later on, however, it produces a harvest of righteousness and peace for those who have been trained by it" (Hebrews 12:11).

"Later on!" We want the harvest now! But discipline is a skill, and skills take time to cultivate.

Learning discipline involves several important factors:

1. *Our relationship to God.*

"My son, do not despise the Lord's discipline and do not resent His rebuke, because the Lord disciplines those He loves, as a father the son he delights in" (Proverbs 3:11–12).

2. *His strength in us.*

"Finally, be strong in the Lord and in His mighty power" (Ephesians 6:10).

3. *New attitudes.*

"You were taught, with regard to your former way of life, to put off your old self, which is being corrupted by its deceitful desires; to be made new in the attitude of your minds; and to put on the new self, created to be like God in true righteousness and holiness" (Ephesians 4:22–24).

4. *New choices.*

"And the peace of God, which transcends all understanding,

will guard your hearts and your minds in Christ Jesus. Finally, brothers, whatever is true, whatever is noble, whatever is right, whatever is pure, whatever is lovely, whatever is admirable—if anything is excellent or praiseworthy—think about such things" (Philippians 4:7–8).

5. *New habits.*

"Do you not know that in a race all the runners run, but only one gets the prize? Run in such a way as to get the prize. Everyone who competes in the games goes into strict training. They do it to get a crown that will not last; but we do it to get a crown that will last forever. Therefore I do not run like a man running aimlessly; I do not fight like a man beating the air. No, I beat my body and make it my slave so that after I have preached to others, I myself will not be disqualified for the prize" (1 Corinthians 9:24–27).

Discipline comes out of recognizing my personal relationship to God (by my choice), His strength working in me (by my choice), adopting new attitudes (by my choice), making new choices (my own), and developing new habits (by my choice). In every regard, I develop discipline because of my own choice.

It's not always fun, it's a challenging responsibility. It's not impossible, but it is hard work. We can't do it apart from God, but He won't do it apart from us; we must choose to be disciplined.

Above all, we have to remember that discipline doesn't start in our behavior; it starts in our mind. The following ten principles will help:

1. *Become aware of God's power in your life.* Place yourself daily in God's hands. Refuse to move in your own strength, but affirm your decision to move only in His.

2. *Consult with God each day about your life.* Moment by moment, learn to "walk in the Lord."

3. *Don't let your mind become careless or slack.*

4. *Refuse to look at the past with regret.* Look to the future with faith.

5. *Feed on the Word of God at every opportunity.*

6. *Be diligent in communion with God.* Pray and praise without ceasing.

7. *Walk in the light of obedience.* The more you obey, the more you'll understand.

8. *Resist the devil with all the spiritual weapons available to*

you. Don't ever treat mental oppression or condemnation as "natural." Fight!

9. *Deal quickly with failure.*

10. *If the enemy breaks through, stand firm.* Don't let him have any more ground, then call your prayer partner for help in recapturing lost territory.

How do you plan to begin to develop the skill of discipline?

_____

_____

_____

How do you plan to incorporate this skill into your life, and when do you plan to begin?

_____

_____

_____

How does seeing discipline as a learned skill differ from how you've seen discipline before?

_____

_____

_____

In what areas are you already applying discipline?

_____

_____

_____

Where do you need to apply it more?

_____

_____

_____

Weekly Evaluation

Goals for the week that I have seen realized:

_____
_____
_____

Goals that were set but only partially realized:

_____
_____
_____

Goals I will carry over to next week because they are worthwhile and important to me:

_____
_____
_____

Goals that I will drop or adjust because they were unrealistic or unimportant:

_____
_____

The most important thing I learned from this week's lesson:

_____
_____
_____

A victory I would like to record:

_____
_____
_____

I am surrendering to God . . .

_____
_____
_____

I am choosing to be more obedient to God in . . .

_____
_____
_____

Overcoming Temptation

Have you ever stayed awake at night wondering why you yielded to a temptation and doubting if you would or could ever change?

Let's be honest. Most of us have.

No matter how strong our resolve or how deep our commitment, all of us have fallen short in maintaining our determination to be strong in the face of temptation at one time or another.

Is there any hope? Yes—hope for every one of us to develop the skill of overcoming temptation. But like discipline, it's a skill that doesn't appear overnight.

Isn't it time you became skillful at overcoming temptation? Do something extraordinary: Become an overcomer. The following five days' quiet times will give you a plan to follow.

✔ Read *The All-New Free to Be Thin*—Chapters 23–24.

Goals for This Week:

- To have a daily quiet time using the Scripture readings assigned.
- To recognize changes I need to make in
  - _____
  - _____
  - _____
- Exercise goal (choose one):
  - ☐ walking _____ minutes per day.
  - ☐ low-impact aerobics class _____ times this week.
  - ☐ low-impact aerobics video tape(title) _____ times this week.

_____
_____
_____

- Other goals:

_____
_____
_____
_____

DAY ONE

READ 1 CORINTHIANS 10:13

THE WAY OUT

God is impressing on me that . . .

I've shared with the Lord that . . .

Thought for the Day:

God doesn't promise escape *from* temptation, but escape in the face of it.

Today's Challenge:

When temptation comes I will face it and look for God's way out.

Food Choices			How Many?	Exchange Group:

Total Exchanges

Bread	Meat	Vegetable	Fruit	Milk	Fat

God is impressing on me that . . .

I've shared with the Lord that . . .

Thought for the Day:

Let's not be strong in our will, but strong in the Lord; not self-sufficient, but drawing from His sufficiency.

Today's Challenge:

I will ask for Christ's help instead of trying to go it alone.

Food Choices				How Many?	Exchange Group:

Total Exchanges

Bread	Meat	Vegetable	Fruit	Milk	Fat

DAY THREE   **READ JOHN 8:31–32**

SPEAK THE TRUTH; ANNOUNCE FREEDOM

God is impressing on me that . . .

I've shared with the Lord that . . .

Thought for the Day:

You can't cherish the freedom if you choke on the truth.

Today's Challenge:

I will walk in truth today and thus experience true freedom.

Food Choices				How Many?	Exchange Group:
Total Exchanges					
Bread	Meat	Vegetable	Fruit	Milk	Fat

God is impressing on me that . . .

I've shared with the Lord that . . .

Thought for the Day:

There are just as many forces to help us avoid sin as there are pressures to give in to it.

Today's Challenge:

I choose to stand in the strength of the Lord and not yield to the pressures of my flesh.

Food Choices				How Many?	Exchange Group:

Total Exchanges

Bread	Meat	Vegetable	Fruit	Milk	Fat

DAY FIVE   **READ ROMANS 8:37**

DECLARE VICTORY!

God is impressing on me that . . .

I've shared with the Lord that . . .

Thought for the Day:

We cannot conquer without the battle.

Today's Challenge:

I acknowledge that I am in a battle but I am victorious in Christ.

Food Choices	How Many?	Exchange Group:

Total Exchanges

Bread	Meat	Vegetable	Fruit	Milk	Fat

LESSON ELEVEN

OVERCOMING TEMPTATION

If you're serious about being a successful Free-to-Be-Thinner, it's because you've accepted the challenge of becoming an overcomer. This skill helps you overcome not only temptations with food but also the temptation to sit when you could exercise, to worry when you could pray, to falter when you could walk steadfast and determined. In other words, an overcoming attitude holds you steady in all of your Christian walk.

Life is strewn with temptations like a field strewn with land mines. Some people grow so afraid to take a step in any direction that they become paralyzed. But that's not what growing Christians do. Instead, they carefully choose each step, and when they see a temptation, they wisely avoid the situation because they have a plan. Here's their strategy:

1. *Look for the way out.*

"No temptation has seized you except what is common to man. And God is faithful; He will not let you be tempted beyond what you can bear. But when you are tempted, He will also provide a way out so that you can stand up under it" (1 Corinthians 10:13).

2. *Ask for Christ's help.*

"Because He himself suffered when He was tempted, He is able to help those who are being tempted" (Hebrews 2:18).

3. *Speak the truth about your situation and announce your freedom.*

"To the Jews who had believed Him, Jesus said, 'If you hold to my teaching, you are really my disciples. Then you will know the truth, and the truth will set you free' " (John 8:31–32).

4. *Proclaim your strength.*

"I can do everything through Him who gives me strength" (Philippians 4:13).

5. *Declare your victory.*

"In all these things we are more than conquerors through Him who loved us" (Romans 8:37).

Henri J. M. Nouwen said this about temptation:

> It may be said that the true quality of the spiritual life can be recognized only in the face of our temptations . . . When we are able to recognize temptations as seductive attempts to make us cling to the illusions of the false self, we can see them as invitations to claim our true self, which is hidden in God and in Him alone.

When we have faced temptations, resisted, and won, Nouwen concludes, "Then we come to know ourselves as God knows us, as sons and daughters, hidden in His love."

The story is told of the rock collector who polished his treasures in a rock tumbler, which jumbles the nuggets together until the rough edges are worn smooth. Someone asked the collector, "How do you know when a rock's been polished enough?"

His answer was simple: "When I can see my reflection in it."

God uses temptation the same way He allows us to be tempted in certain areas of our life until He can see His reflection. When the testing is complete, we will desire God alone.

Falling into temptations, facing various testings and trials, are a part of the normal Christian life. But those times can be valuable opportunities for growth and strengthening—*if* we see them in light of our transformation into the image of Jesus Christ.

Remember, temptation is not a sin, nor is it a sign of certain failure. Instead, it's the work of a loving God giving us an opportunity to grow. Remember, too, that with temptation, God has a plan. Use it!

Answer the following questions:

In your own words, describe the difference between being tempted and falling into temptation:

_____
_____
_____

Why should you expect not to be exempt from temptation or trial?

_____
_____
_____

What can times of temptation show you?

_____

_____

What difference does this lesson make to you in your daily walk
with Christ?

_____

_____

In your attitude toward temptation?

_____

_____

_____

WEEKLY EVALUATION

Goals for the week that I have seen realized:

_____

_____

_____

Goals that were set but only partially realized:

_____

_____

_____

Goals I will carry over to next week because they are worthwhile
and important to me:

_____

_____

_____

Goals that I will drop or adjust because they were unrealistic or
unimportant:

_____

_____

The most important thing I learned from this week's lesson:

_____

_____

_____

A victory I would like to record:

_____

_____

_____

I am surrendering to God . . .

_____

_____

_____

I am choosing to be more obedient to God in . . .

_____

_____

_____

PERSEVERANCE

Have you ever wanted to quit? Maybe you've worked hard on some project or on some area of your life, only to have things backfire. Worse yet, you're the one who got burned.

Maybe it's happened since you began this study. With all the effort you could muster, you've tried to grow, to handle the situations that have come up in light of your new insights, only to discover that even though you've grown, you haven't grown enough. What's worse, the growth was painful, and it's evident that further pain lies ahead.

At times like that, it's tempting just to quit. Give it all up. Check out. I know, because I've been at that place myself. I understand what it's like not only to want to quit, but to feel as if there's no other choice.

We can list all kinds of reasons, seemingly good reasons, for wanting the world to stop so we can get off. We may even pray for the soon return of the Lord—all the while afraid for it to happen because of the spiritual state we're in.

What it really boils down to is this: In the face of troubles, we lose sight of the purpose and victory we want to see in our lives. We're confronted with a choice to *go on* or *get off*, and we don't feel as if we can go on.

Nevertheless, God calls us to be disciplined overcomers, not quitters. When things are hardest, when we're the least motivated to go on, we hear Him whispering, *"Persevere."*

When quitting seems the easiest route and perseverance, the hardest; when the challenge has long ago lost its excitement; when the discipline is no longer fresh, but routine—that's when we need perseverance the most.

Perseverance is not what *characterizes* mature Christians; it's what produces them.

That's why the apostle Paul didn't list perseverance as a fruit of the Spirit—something you grow naturally. Instead, it's a skill produced through discipline and practice.

How do we learn perseverance? The Scripture readings we'll examine this week show us how.

▶ Read *The All-New Free to Be Thin*—Chapters 25–26.

GOALS FOR THIS WEEK:

- To have a daily quiet time using the Scripture readings assigned.
- To recognize changes I need to make in
    - _____
    - _____
    - _____
- Exercise goal (choose one):
    ☐ walking _____ minutes per day.
    ☐ low-impact aerobics class _____ times this week.
    ☐ low-impact aerobics video tape(title) _____ times this week.

_____
_____
_____

- Other goals:

_____
_____
_____
_____

DAY ONE   **READ JAMES 1:2-4**

CONSIDER IT JOY!

God is impressing on me that . . .

I've shared with the Lord that . . .

Thought for the Day:

How we define our troubles and testings determines whether or not we can see God's hand in our circumstances.

Today's Challenge:

Today I will consider it all joy when I come up against a test.

Food Choices	How Many?	Exchange Group:
Total Exchanges		

Bread	Meat	Vegetable	Fruit	Milk	Fat

God is impressing on me that . . .

I've shared with the Lord that . . .

Thought for the Day:

Jesus knows what it's like to face a crisis. He saw beyond the cross, beyond the rejection, beyond the emotional and physical pain to the purpose God had for Him.

Today's Challenge:

When faced with a painful circumstance, I will be much more likely to look beyond the moment to the purpose.

Food Choices	How Many?	Exchange Group:

Total Exchanges

Bread	Meat	Vegetable	Fruit	Milk	Fat

God is impressing on me that . . .

I've shared with the Lord that . . .

Thought for the Day:

Right now—this very day, this very hour, in the middle of this very trying circumstance—I have the opportunity to learn to persevere.

Today's Challenge:

I choose to be full of hope.

Food Choices				How Many?	Exchange Group:

Total Exchanges

Bread	Meat	Vegetable	Fruit	Milk	Fat

HOLD ON!

God is impressing on me that . . .

I've shared with the Lord that . . .

Thought for the Day:

The Christian life is not guaranteed to be easy. But we *can* be made equal to the challenges; we *can* persevere.

Today's Challenge:

I will look for an opportunity to persevere today.

Food Choices	How Many?	Exchange Group:

Total Exchanges

Bread	Meat	Vegetable	Fruit	Milk	Fat

GO ON!

God is impressing on me that . . .

I've shared with the Lord that . . .

Thought for the Day:

Perseverance isn't found only in the life of those who are "victorious" or "successful," but also in the life of those who stumble and fail—as long as they keep trying, pick themselves up, and go on.

Today's Challenge:

I resolve to go on in the face of difficulty.

Food Choices	How Many?	Exchange Group:

Total Exchanges

Bread	Meat	Vegetable	Fruit	Milk	Fat

PERSEVERANCE

Right now—this very day, this very hour, in the middle of this very trying circumstance—is when you must learn to persevere. It's the toughest skill you may ever have to cultivate as a Christian, perhaps even the hardest challenge you've ever undertaken. But if being made into the image of Jesus Christ is a priority in your life, then a perseverer you must become.

No doubt we all prefer life without complications: no storms, no clouds, no pests, no tests. An environment of peace, tranquility, and comfort sounds wonderful. But that's not reality. This isn't heaven; it's earth, and while we remain in it we'll have struggles.

It helps to remember that we're not the only ones to find that life has hard places. Everyone does. The Christian life isn't guaranteed to be easy. But we *can* be made equal to the challenges. We can persevere.

Perseverance isn't found only in the life of those who are "victorious" or "successful," but also in the life of those who stumble and fail—as long as they keep trying, picking themselves up, and going on. Perseverance isn't gained in the absence of failure, but in the face of it.

Successful perseverers have learned to do five important things:

1. *They consider it joy.*

"Consider it pure joy, my brothers, whenever you face trials of many kinds, because you know that the testing of your faith develops perseverance. Perseverance must finish its work so that you may be mature and complete, not lacking anything" (James 1:2–4).

2. *They look to Jesus.*

"Therefore, since we are surrounded by such a great cloud of witnesses, let us throw off everything that hinders and the sin that so easily entangles, and let us run with perseverance the race marked out for us. Let us fix our eyes on Jesus, the author and perfecter of our faith, who for the joy set before Him endured the cross, scorning its shame, and sat down at the right hand of the throne of God" (Hebrews 12:1-2).

3. *They maintain hope.*

"But if we hope for what we do not yet have, we wait for it patiently" (Romans 8:25).

4. *They hold on.*

"You need to persevere so that when you have done the will of God, you will receive what He has promised. For in just a very little while, 'He who is coming will come and will not delay. But my righteous one will live by faith. And if he shrinks back, I will not be pleased with him.' But we are not of those who shrink back and are destroyed, but of those who believe and are saved" (Hebrews 10:36-39).

5. *They go on.*

"Keep me safe, O God, for in you I take refuge. I said to the LORD, 'You are my Lord; apart from you I have no good thing' " (Psalm 16:1-2).

"The boundary lines have fallen for me in pleasant places; surely I have a delightful inheritance. I will praise the LORD, who counsels me; even at night my heart instructs me. I have set the LORD always before me. Because He is at my right hand, I will not be shaken. Therefore my heart is glad and my tongue rejoices; my body also will rest secure" (Psalm 16:6-9).

Think of it: If you could instantly replace all illness with health, poverty with prosperity, anger and hurt with joy and forgiveness, how would you grow? How would you cultivate compassion? Tolerance? How would your character develop?

Remember that there's a work going on inside Christians. We're being disciplined and shaped into the image of Jesus Christ (see Philippians 1:6). Christians don't live without trouble and tests, but they've been given the power to become overcomers and to grow through the struggles of life. Yet this marvelous opportunity comes only through perseverance.

Perseverance is what matures us and completes us so that we're not lacking anything (see James 1:4). It makes us whole in Christ, with nothing left out. Trials and temptations coming at us full force only cause us to develop a perseverance that carries each of us through, all the while developing the perfection of Christ in us.

What situations in your life right now irritate or antagonize you?

_____

_____

_____

What changes need to be made in your attitudes before God can use these circumstances to bring forth the perfect work He wants to do in you?

_____

_____

_____

What changes in your prayers do you need to make before God can bring about desired changes in you?

_____

_____

_____

How can you tell whether you trust God to know what's best for you?

_____

_____

_____

If you're brave enough, write a prayer that God will do a work in you to develop perseverance:

_____

_____

_____

_____

If He were to answer your prayer, how do you think He would do it?

_____

_____

_____

WEEKLY EVALUATION

Goals for the week that I have seen realized:

_____
_____
_____

Goals that were set but only partially realized:

_____
_____
_____

Goals I will carry over to next week because they are worthwhile
and important to me:

_____
_____
_____

Goals that I will drop or adjust because they were unrealistic or
unimportant:

_____
_____

The most important thing I learned from this week's lesson:

_____
_____
_____

A victory I would like to record:

_____
_____
_____

I am surrendering to God . . .

_____
_____
_____

I am choosing to be more obedient to God in . . .

_____
_____
_____

Rest

"This is what the Sovereign LORD, the Holy One of Israel, says: 'In repentance and rest is your salvation, in quietness and trust is your strength' " (Isaiah 30:15).

I suppose we could end this study with a strong pep talk on how I believe you can do it—and I do believe that. Or I could try to pump you up one more time for another strong urge of determination and try to drag further commitments of obedience from you. But I believe you need something quite different at this point. You need rest.

Are you experienced in rest? Do you know what it actually is to cease from work, from activity, and from going through the motions? Do you know the peace that comes from genuine quietness, or do you only know how to be busy doing something, *anything*, that keeps you moving in what you think is the right direction?

In chapter 12 we said to go on and not give up; now we're saying to rest. Is there a contradiction here? No. Rest isn't giving up; it's simply finding relief and freedom. It's being refreshed, free from anxiety or distress.

This isn't the same as stopping. Instead, it means that we finally find repose in Christ, peace with God, and joy in who we are in Him. We come to realize God's promise as He first spoke it to Moses: "My presence will go with you, and I will give you rest" (Exodus 33:14).

The peaceful rest that God promises His children is not the same as catching your breath or taking a break. Rather, it's a time with Him when you focus more on the Master than on the task, more on the Savior than on the challenge. This is where we find mental and even physical recuperation. It's where we discover peace of mind, complete absence of worry or weariness of effort. It's the place of comfort, well-being, and satisfaction.

No matter what you weighed at the beginning of this study,

or what you weigh now at the end, you can have this rest. Thinness doesn't give it to us; Jesus does. It's not something you qualify for—it's something He wants to give you. Will you let Him?

GOALS FOR THIS WEEK:

- To have a daily quiet time using the Scripture readings assigned.
- To recognize changes I need to make in
    - _____
    - _____
    - _____
- Exercise goal (choose one):
  ☐ walking _____ minutes per day.
  ☐ low-impact aerobics class _____ times this week.
  ☐ low-impact aerobics video tape (title) _____ times this week.

  _____
  _____
  _____

- Other goals:

  _____
  _____
  _____
  _____

DAY ONE   **READ MATTHEW 11:28**

REST FROM THE STRUGGLE.

God is impressing on me that . . .

I've shared with the Lord that . . .

Thought for the Day:

We often want to learn the gentle lessons from Christ while trying to negotiate the yoke.

Today's Challenge:

I choose to take on Christ's yoke today.

Food Choices	How Many?	Exchange Group:

Total Exchanges

Bread	Meat	Vegetable	Fruit	Milk	Fat

REST IN HIS LOVE.

God is impressing on me that . . .

I've shared with the Lord that . . .

Thought for the Day:

It's not because of us that our mistakes aren't fatal, but because of His love.

Today's Challenge:

I will truly rest in His love and His ability to keep me from falling.

Food Choices	How Many?	Exchange Group:

Total Exchanges

Bread	Meat	Vegetable	Fruit	Milk	Fat

DAY THREE   **READ PSALM 23**

REST IN HIS CARE.

God is impressing on me that...

I've shared with the Lord that...

Thought for the Day:

God knows exactly what we need and when we need it. It's not for us to press for the answer to our need, but to press in to Him.

Today's Challenge:

In the face of need or want I will rest in Him.

Food Choices	How Many?	Exchange Group:

Total Exchanges

Bread	Meat	Vegetable	Fruit	Milk	Fat

DAY FOUR   **READ EXODUS 33:14**

REST IN HIS PRESENCE.

God is impressing on me that . . .

I've shared with the Lord that . . .

Thought for the Day:

Why would God promise us His presence if He thought we could make it on our own?

Today's Challenge:

I admit I can't do it alone.

Food Choices	How Many?	Exchange Group:

Total Exchanges

Bread	Meat	Vegetable	Fruit	Milk	Fat

DAY FIVE   **READ 1 CORINTHIANS 15:58**
REST IN SUBMISSION.

God is impressing on me that . . .

I've shared with the Lord that . . .

Thought for the Day:

God is doing a far greater work in our hearts than He is in our bodies.

Today's Challenge:

I believe that God is working in me in spite of any physical evidence.

Food Choices	How Many?	Exchange Group:

Total Exchanges

Bread	Meat	Vegetable	Fruit	Milk	Fat

REST

"Come here," Jesus says to us. "I want to give you something."

"What is it, Lord?"

"Rest."

"But Lord, I haven't reached my goal yet. I'm still above 190 pounds. Later, Lord—once I've broken the 160-pound barrier. Then I'll rest."

"Now," says the Lord. "I want to give you rest *now*."

"But Jesus," we protest, "if I stop to rest now, I'll lose my momentum. I might not be able to start again. Not now, Lord. I can't rest now."

Sound familiar? I've certainly had mental conversations like this with Jesus myself. And looking back, I can see that my excuses for not resting were all based on one assumption: We can't rest until the job is done. Only those who have finished the course and met the goal can rest.

When we base our understanding of rest on God's Word however, His invitation to rest not only makes good sense—it moves us toward our goal even faster. Why is that? Because rest gives us more strength to carry out our responsibilities.

We sometimes get the feeling that "rest" means taking a break or abandoning all responsibility. Yet we're not talking here about resting *from* our responsibilities, but resting *in* them. We don't rest *from* obedience; we rest *in* it. We don't rest *from* the daily quiet time, but *in* it. We don't rest *from* prayer, but *in* it.

In the last three months, you've learned new principles and practices. You've been busy developing new habits through discipline and perseverance. Now it's time to rest—not *from* what you've been doing, but *in* it.

Hear Jesus whisper: "Come to me, all you who are weary and burdened, and I will give you rest." You still have responsibility, and He says: "Take my yoke upon you and learn from me." But you will nevertheless "find rest for your soul" (Matthew 11:28). That means you'll rest *from* the struggle and rest *from* self-effort, even while you rest *in* His yoke and rest *in* Him. Here's how:

1. *Rest in His love.* Let the truth sink deep within your spirit that *nothing* can separate you from Christ's love (see Romans 8:35–39). Nothing you can ever do will make Him love you any more or any less. He loves you—that's settled. So rest in it.

2. *Rest in His care.* Read the twenty-third Psalm as many times as you need to, to understand that He cares for you—that He will take care of you. "The Lord will fulfill His purpose for me," says Psalm 138:8. Will you rest in His care?

3. *Rest in His presence* (see Exodus 33:14). He is here—here for you.

How do you rest? By faith. By faith, food issues become settled issues once and for all. By faith, weight issues are resolved in His love, in His care, and in His presence. By faith, our responsibilities continue, of course, but in His provision and in light of the love He has for us.

Finally, as you rest, "stand firm. Let nothing move you. Always give yourselves fully to the work of the Lord, because you know that your labor in the Lord is not in vain" (1 Corinthians 15:58). Give yourself fully to the work the Lord is doing *in* you as well as the work He wants to do *through* you. Be stubborn in your rest even as you're stubborn in your submission to the work He wants to do in you.

When you see commercials offering questionable weight-loss products, stand firm. Don't be moved. *Rest.*

When you see friends doing all kinds of crazy things to lose weight—and with apparent success—stand firm. *Rest.*

When others ask you if you're still on a diet, *rest.*

When it takes a long time and you have to persevere to a degree you've never known before, *rest.* Simply believe God, and rest.

Resting in Jesus Christ will give you full protection from discouragement. He is your haven. Let Him shelter you from shame and feelings of futility. Find in Him an assurance of His love and care.

You'll never again have to worry about your weight. In Christ you're *doing* something about it: You're submitting to new principles, walking in new truths, developing new habits, all the while resting in Him.

Does this all sound too good to be true? What have you got

to lose by trusting in God? Put your faith to the test. You won't be disappointed.

This is your moment, a turning point of your life. The issues of food and weight management can be settled once and for all. You've got what it takes—Jesus in you.

Answer the following questions:

What difference has the past thirteen-week study made in you?

_____

_____

_____

_____

How do you view your weight differently from the way you did at the beginning?

_____

_____

_____

How do you plan to continue the work begun in you through this study?

_____

_____

_____

Based on what you sensed God speaking to you during your quiet times these past weeks, write out a simple statement of commitment to peace and rest:

_____

_____

_____

_____

EVALUATION

During this study, I've made positive changes in the following areas:

_____ attitudes toward myself

_____ food habits and choices

_____ consistent exercise routine

_____ daily quiet time

_____ attitudes toward others

I've seen the following prayers answered:

_____

_____

_____

_____

Other goals I've seen realized:

_____

_____

_____

_____

My weight today: _____ My eating habits have improved in these ways:

_____ better control

_____ fewer binges

_____ better food choices

_____ other: _____

I find myself

_____ enjoying discipline in my life

_____ free from extremes and obsessions concerning food and diets

_____ able to ask for help and support when I need it to maintain consistency

Changes I've made that I'm confident are permanent:

_____

_____

Changes I've made that are still quite fragile and still need support:

Going on from here means:

GROUP GUIDELINE SUGGESTIONS AND LEADER'S NOTES

This study may be used in several ways. The first is to make it a personal devotional study without help from a leader or a group. The second is to work through it with a partner or in a neighborhood Bible study group with planned discussion questions and prayer time. A third option is to adapt this material for an already existing group such as a Sunday school class.

Whether used privately or in a group setting, this study will take thirteen weeks to complete. Each part of the book is designed to be worked through individually during the week between meetings so that insights can be shared and questions discussed at the meeting. Sample discussion questions are included in the Leader's Notes.

GETTING STARTED

If you're interested in beginning a group study of this material, consider these steps toward that goal:

1. Pray!

2. Talk with your pastor about beginning a group in your church congregation. We encourage interested individuals or groups to meet the needs of overweight people by using this concept in the context of the local church, because that's the primary place where such ministry should be occurring. Of course, it's vital that the leaders of the group be in good standing with the local church and have the approval and support of their senior pastor.

3. Find others to join your group through a notice in your church bulletin or an announcement posted on a church bulletin board or in your local Christian bookstore.

4. Set a date for an initial orientation session for interested people.

5. To begin, each person will need a copy of *The All-New Free to Be Thin* by Neva Coyle and Marie Chapian (Bethany House Publishers, 1993) and a copy of this journal. You can order them for the whole group through your local Christian bookstore. Be sure to ask how long it will take for the materials to arrive, then allow enough time between your orientation and your first meeting.

Please note: It is illegal for any group other than Overeaters Victorious, Inc., to use the protected corporate name on any bank account or advertising materials. The material produced and published by and for this ministry is copyrighted and cannot be reproduced in any form without express written permission. Funds of local groups are the sole responsibility of the local leader or sponsoring church.

GENERAL GUIDELINES FOR THE GROUP LEADER

Personal investigation followed by shared responses make the best study approach for a group. Discussion questions will help uncover even more insights into application for personal growth.

Since the material covered may delve into some sensitive and private matters, don't force or even expect everyone to participate in every meeting. Encourage even the slightest participation with affirmative comments, regardless of the contribution. There are no wrong answers in this study.

You'll be getting to the heart of several emotional issues in the process. For that reason, some people in your group may desperately need a listening ear; others may be so sensitive that a minor correction from you could discourage them from participating in your discussions or even attending your group. Allow the Holy Spirit to do the correction in them and a deep work of patience and sensitivity in you.

If some individual monopolizes the conversation or goes off on a tangent, carefully approach that person afterward and ask whether you can be of help individually. Of course, there will be those days when people genuinely come to a "breakthrough" and will consequently draw the attention of the group to themselves and their needs exclusively. That should be the exception, however, and not the rule.

When someone in your group asks a question, allow others to respond before you do. You don't have to be the one with all the answers, and you'll find yourself learning as much as everyone else.

There are only three basic rules that you should strive to keep without fail:

1. *Start and end on time.* Everyone is busy, so don't waste anyone's time. Set your meeting times and stick to them. One and a half hours works well for evening groups, while daytime groups can meet a little longer. Actual study discussion will only take a portion of that time. Having fellowship and sharing prayer requests helps develop strong bonds within your group, so make time for that to happen as well.

2. *Begin and end with prayer.* Opening prayer time can be simple: Just have one person ask God's blessing on your time together, much like asking the blessing before a meal. You might also want to have a time to pray for concerns beyond the group. One effective way to handle this need is to have each group member write down on a slip of paper the name of the person he or she is concerned for, along with a brief statement of the need. The slips are put into a basket and redistributed to the group. Each person then says a one-sentence prayer for the person whose need he or she has drawn from the basket.

Closing prayers can be centered on the group members' needs related to the study and the discussion questions. Waiting until all those who wish to pray have done so, and then offering a final prayer is a good way for leaders to bring the meeting to a close.

3. *Involve everyone.* Many of the issues addressed in this study are sensitive. Given the abuse and misunderstanding many of your group members have experienced, they may not be ready to discuss the issues they're dealing with right away. However, fellowship time, prayer for others, and other group activities will build trust and help them to open up and share. Find a way to involve even the most reserved members in a way that is comfortable and safe for them.

LEADER'S NOTES FOR LESSON ONE

Briefly have each person share a defeat he or she experienced this week. At this point, don't give advice or bring the discussion to a conclusion; that will come later.

Read together Luke 15:11.

Discussion questions:

1. What are some of the ways in which we all stray from the Father's care and protection?
2. What encouragement do you get from the words, "I will arise and go to my Father"?
3. What decision does that encourage us to make?
4. Tell about a victory from this week's bold new beginning.
5. Share your favorite "Food Supplement" and tell why it's your favorite.
6. Rephrase the description of your defeat into a prayer request.
7. Rephrase the description of your defeat into a goal for next week.

End with prayer for each person in the group, praying specifically about the requests and for strength to meet the goals.

LEADER'S NOTES FOR LESSON TWO

Group members should have completed the questionnaire in Appendix B.

Discussion questions:

1. Weight-loss history is essential to each person's success—or lack of it. It is now known that each weight-loss experience, followed by weight regain, makes losing and maintaining a weight loss much more difficult. What has been your experience in this regard?
2. What are some of the ways a weight regain might affect a person?
3. Exercise is essential not only to a weight-loss program, but also to a person's overall health. Yet overweight people tend to drop out of exercise routines. Why?
4. What hobbies contribute to a sedentary lifestyle? How can we change that?
5. How can trauma be associated with weight gain or loss?
6. What does the way we handle emergencies have to do with overeating?
7. How are overeating and emotions connected?
8. What adjustments must we make to our approach if we don't have a supportive spouse during this time of change?
9. What thoughts do you have about getting an OV partner? Have

you considered who would make a good partner for you? Who is it, and why do you think this person will make a good prayer partner?

10. What kind of OV partner would you make? Why do you think so?

11. Did any unexpected attitudes surface while answering the "Questions to Consider" in Appendix C? Comments:

Read to the group the following quote from *We Really Do Need Each Other* by Reuben Welch[1]:

> The life that Jesus brings is a shared life. The life of God in the world does not have its meaning in isolated units, but in a fellowship of those who share that life in Him.
>
> Christians are not brought together because they like each other, but because they share a common life in Jesus and are faced with the task of learning how to love each other as members of the family. . . .
>
> The church is not the society of the congenial—it is a fellowship based on common life in Jesus. It is the will of God that the Christian life be lived in the context of a fellowship of the shared life. God has made us in such a way that we really do need each other.
>
> Some of us are so westernized and individualized and evangelicalized that we have forgotten how much we really need each other. I think people like you and me are grossly over-individualized. I think we have talked about personal salvation and individual salvation and "me" and "my" and "my inner life" until we have almost isolated ourselves. And so we just get the idea that it's my life, and God's life and you have your relationship to God and I have my relationship to God and of course we ought to love each other, but what really counts is "my relationship to God."
>
> We Christians act as though we are deep sea divers. Here we are in the murky waters of sin—but we have the protection of the diving suit of God and we have the lifeline that goes to the great white ship up above. You have your life in Christ, and your lifeline, and I have my life in Christ and my lifeline, and here we are with all our lifelines going up. And we say to each other, "How's your lifeline, brother—any kinks? Get it straightened out, keep the oxygen going, or the

---

[1]Taken from the book *We Really Do Need Each Other*, by Reuben Welch. Copyright © 1973 by Impact Books. Used by permission of Zondervan Publishing House.

murky waters of sin will come rushing in on you."

We wave to each other and write notes to each other and we bump each other around and we say to each other—"Get your lifeline right."

But here I am, all by myself. Once in a while someone gets the bends and we bump him to the top or just cut him off and let him drown. That's not the way it is, because our life that we have with God is not just my life and His—no way.

I know this vertical relationship is fundamental. I know what constitutes us as a community is His life given. I'm not saying that our relationship to God is not personal and unique. I'm saying we are over-individualized.

The vertical line of God-ward relationship and the horizontal line of human relationship are not two lines but one line in a continuum. It all belongs together. I'm not talking about what ought to be or what would be nice if it were— I'm talking about the way He constituted the life we have with Him. Our life with Him is tied to, is one with our life with our brothers and sisters.

When we feel like we are slipping spiritually or growing cold or indifferent we have a tendency to withdraw and pray through or to get hold of God or get back to where we ought to be so we will have something to give to others—and that's false.

That separates the full and the empty, the haves and the have-nots. But on our own, outside of Christ, we are all *have-nots*, we are all *emptys*.

I have heard it said, "Real witnessing is one beggar telling another beggar where to get bread." We are all beggars—we don't have anything but the life of Christ, and His life in us is not separate from our life with each other.

I think we are helped in this feeling of isolation by the songs that we sing:

When I am burdened
    or weary or sad,
Jesus is all I need.

or,

    Are you weary;
      are you heavy-hearted;
    tell it to Jesus alone.

Of course there is truth in all these songs. Of course we believe in the total adequacy of Jesus Christ to meet the total need of the total person.

But we must remember this also—He saves in the context

of the community of faith. It isn't "Jesus and me" it is "Jesus and we" and on the Jericho Road there is room for Jesus and the whole redeemed community. And if you are like me, when you are burdened and weary and sad you need Jesus but you also need someone to be Jesus to you—someone to bring His healing presence to you.

Sometimes the answer to your weariness and heavy-heartedness is not to "tell it to Jesus alone" but to begin to share and care with someone else.

You see, we really do need each other, not because of the inadequacies of God, but because this is the way His grace works.

And I tell you this—if somewhere in the world there are people who are sharing the life of Jesus together and who are helping each other, and suffering with each other, that's my crowd. Those are the people—that is the community of which my heart yearns to be a part. And the name of it is the Church, the body of Christ, the fellowship of believers.

Read the introduction to Lesson Three together and compute calorie needs for safe weight loss. Discuss food ideas and the exchange plan.

Pray together.

LEADER'S NOTES FOR LESSON THREE

Discussion questions:
1. What is your reaction to the higher calorie limits?
2. If taking the time for your metabolism to correct itself meant a temporary weight gain, how would you react?
3. What difference does it make to your attitude toward the scale to know that these lessons are about a covenant relationship with God—not about obeying a set of rules?
4. If obedient actions are an expression of a covenant relationship with God, how is that reflected on your daily quiet time sheets and food diaries?
5. Looking over your food choices, what things do you need to eat more of? What items would it be wise to eat less of?
6. How can your partner be of more help to you?
7. Tell about a sabotage experience. Tell about a support experience.
8. What was the most important thing you learned from Lesson Three?
9. Share your favorite verse from this lesson.

LEADER'S NOTES FOR LESSON FOUR

In this lesson it's especially important for you as the group leader to plant the week's scriptural principles deep into your own heart. Your group will need extra encouragement from you at this critical time. To help you minister an extra dose of God's love, power, and purpose, the following exercise is essential.

Have on hand three different versions of the Bible (for example, the *New American Standard*, the *New International Version*, and the *New King James Bible*). Settle your group into an atmosphere of contemplation and quietness. Then read aloud, slowly, from one version, Haggai 1:8, 2:3–9 as a single passage, letting the full message of the passage sink in. Without any discussion or words spoken in the group, have each person write a few thoughts on the page provided in chapter four. (page 80.)

After a few moments, read the same passage from another version. Again, without verbal response, have each one respond in writing.

Finally, read the passage a third time from the third version. After you read, pause for a few moments, then open it up to discussion about the impact of this passage.

Discussion questions:

1. When you review your calorie limit and your food choices of this past week in light of these five biblical principles, how does your perspective change on previous attempts at weight or over-eating management?

2. What is your reaction to a longer, slower approach to change and weight or overeating management?

3. What changes are you seeing take place in
your attitudes? _____
your eating or good choices? _____
other aspects of your life that seem unrelated, yet are also being affected by this study? _____

LEADER'S NOTES FOR LESSON FIVE

Tell the group some of the ways in which you've seen God work in your heart since the beginning of this study in an area that has nothing to do with losing or gaining weight.

Ask them to do the same.

Discussion questions:

1. What are some of the ways in which you sense that God's work

in you is directly related to your weight or eating habits?

2. What has been the most beneficial biblical principle you have learned so far, and why?

3. How have this week's five biblical principles helped you get ready to weigh?

Pray before weighing together.

Talk over the victories and the defeats. Be sensitive to the one who has lost the least and ask what God is doing in her or him, regardless of the lack of weight loss.

Read Philippians 2:1-4 aloud together and discuss ways to keep one another's interests in focus and perspective.

LEADER'S NOTES FOR LESSON SIX

Read Daniel 1 aloud in class (from *The Amplified Version of the Bible*, if possible).

Discussion questions:

1. Daniel knew he was chosen for the king's personal service, yet he chose to obey only God. Why?

2. What clue does the Scripture give about the source of Daniel's strength to obey God rather than the king's orders?

3. How did God honor Daniel's decision to obey only Him?

4. What was the result?

5. Read aloud together 2 Corinthians 5:14-21. Which king have you been chosen to obey and serve?

6. How can Daniel serve as an example for you?

7. What decisions have you come to about a renewed commitment?

8. How can you confirm your decisions?

Conclude with prayers for strength and courage to live out your renewed commitments.

LEADER'S NOTES FOR LESSON SEVEN

Take some time to talk over exercise experiences. Let each person express personal preferences as to type, duration, effectiveness.

Desires/Actions Worksheet

Together, create a Desires/Actions Worksheet, using a large poster on which you have copied the format shown below. Transfer the worksheet onto an overhead transparency and project the chart on a wall or screen.

Desires/Actions Worksheet

Psalm 37:4: "Delight yourself in the Lord, and He will give you the desires of your heart."

DESIRES	ACTIONS
Psalm 27:4: "One thing have I desired from the Lord . . .	. . . that will I seek after."
Date	Date

Have someone in the class read Psalm 27:4 (KJV), calling attention to the two phrases, "One thing have I desired," and "that will I seek after."

Discussion questions:

1. Often what we say we desire is not reflected in our choices. For example, we may say we want to lose weight yet we eat a high-fat, low-fiber diet. We may insist that we want to exercise yet never get around to doing it. In this way we sabotage our desires. What are some other ways that we sabotage our desires?

2. How can some of the desires we've written on the chart be sabotaged?

3. How does setting goals and evaluating each week help us fulfill our desires?

4. Recall an experience in which you spotted a potential self-sabotage coming and averted it.

After this discussion, have each person take a few moments to fill out his or her own Desires/Actions Worksheet.

End the class session by talking over desires and rephrasing them into prayers.

LEADER'S NOTES FOR LESSON EIGHT

Discussion questions:

1. When Jesus called the first disciple He said, "Follow me and I will make you . . ." (Matthew 4:19, KJV).

In those few words He reveals that He can take us as we are and help us to become what He sees we can be. What changes do you see God making in you?

2. Read Jeremiah 31:31–37 aloud. What part of this passage helped you to resist temptation this week? Tell about a specific example.

What part of this passage helped you to overcome a failure this week? Be specific.

What part of this passage helps you to look at your relationship to God differently than you did before? How?

3. In a few words, give your definition of the new thing you are experiencing with regard to your weight, attitudes, habits, and other areas of your life.

4. How can we redefine the struggles we're presently experiencing in light of the concept of God's "new thing"? Be specific.

Close with prayer.

LEADER'S NOTES FOR LESSON NINE

Discussion questions:

1. How can it be that we do not experience the reality of our position in Christ moment by moment?

2. When do you feel the most insecure?

3. How does knowing your security in Christ help you to change how you deal with insecurity?

4. Look at the graph on page 167 of this lesson, and tell us where your experience stands right now.

5. What is your true position in Christ?

6. Which line expresses the reality of our position in Christ? Which line expresses the reality of our present experience?

7. Are there personal dangers for you in acting on a lesson like this one?

8. How do you plan to avoid those dangers?

9. When do we grow most—during times of ease or times of challenge? Why?

10. How can we best pray for one another in light of the truth of this lesson?

LEADER'S NOTES FOR LESSON TEN

Discussion questions:

1. Discuss the difference between a characteristic and a skill. Use a dictionary if necessary.

2. Review together the ten principles of discipline and have the group discuss any additional insights they've gained in applying them to eating patterns and food choices.

3. Rephrase each of the ten principles of discipline as goals.

4. Which of the ten principles of discipline would you like to rephrase into a prayer request?

LEADER'S NOTES FOR LESSON ELEVEN

Discussion questions:
1. Have you made a firm commitment before the Lord to obedience and faithfulness concerning a particular issue in your life? Tell us about that commitment.
2. How was that commitment tested? Name some of the temptations that tested it.
3. Remember an occasion when you faced temptation and chose to overcome. How did that affect you and your walk with the Lord?
4. What temptation(s) are you struggling with at the present?
5. What do you think is God's will concerning these temptations?
6. How can you state your struggle as a prayer request?

LEADER'S NOTES FOR LESSON TWELVE

Discussion questions:
1. In your own words, define "perseverance."
2. Why is it God's will to develop perseverance in us?
3. How will He most likely do this?
4. In his book *Adventure in Adversity* [2], Paul Billheimer says: "[God] is more interested in spiritual health and maturity than He is in temporary physical comfort. In all of His dealing with us, God is working toward greater holiness."

How has this study been used by God to develop you into a stronger, more mature Christian?
5. Paul Billheimer also says: "In our own way, each of us who yields his life unreservedly into the hands of God, finds himself passing through the various stages, experiences, and discoveries concerning suffering through which Job passed. He finally reached a point where he could begin to understand something of the purpose of his afflictions. Although perfect in a relative sense, he still needed further discipline; he still needed refinement. And most of us do also. This viewpoint is often overlooked. Too many of us who feel that we are mature in grace fail to realize that God may yet have a controversy with something in our character or personality and that there may remain graces of the Spirit which God can add to us only through affliction.

---

[2]Published by Trinity Broadcasting Network.

"We may need to remember that no matter how we may be, there are new heights and new depths of grace, new graces and virtues that await a new revelation of God."[3]

How would you apply this insight to your particular circumstances?

6. What are the qualities of the Christian walk that you see God developing in you through perseverance?

7. In his book *No Substitute for Persevering*,[4] Reuben Welch says: "We have tasted the 'heavenly gift', but live in the real world where we know both joy and sorrow, victory and defeat. Sometimes it is just fantastic, but at other times we run out of fantastic and grow weary on the way. At such times we need to know again that Jesus, our Priest and Brother, is with us where we are and strengthens us by His spirit to persevere."

How is Jesus helping you to persevere?

8. Of the three skills we've noted—discipline, overcoming temptation, and perseverance—which is the most difficult for you? Why?

9. If we become disciplined overcomers who know how to persevere, how will that change our lives?

10. What else is needed to be successful in our weight management or to control overeating?

LEADER'S NOTES FOR LESSON THIRTEEN

Review again together the questions in Appendix C. This time, have the group write their answers in column B. Note how the group's answers after the completion of the study differ from those at the beginning.

Review the reasons for weighing as outlined in Lesson Five and discuss feelings about weighing. When everyone is ready, weigh, and then add the weight losses together. Thank God as a group for the total weight lost to His glory. Be sure to emphasize that any individual's victory also belongs to the entire group.

Small awards or special recognition could be given to those who

_____ came every week.

_____ were successful in their five quiet times each week.

---

[3]*Don't Waste Your Sorrows*, Bethany House Publishers, 1977.
[4]Published by Zondervan, 1982.

_____ were faithful to their prayer partner commitment.
Let the group select
_____ the one showing the greatest change in attitudes.
_____ the one who deserves recognition for being an encourager.
_____ the one who showed the most determination in the face of difficulties during the past thirteen weeks.
Close this special day with the following prayer:

Dear Father, Thank you for loving us. Thank you for showing us how much You love and care for each one of us, and that You understand the pressures we've been under that have tempted us to harm our bodies. Thank you for helping us to be free from obsessions with food and with dieting. Thank you for showing us a purpose for life apart from food and diets. Thank you, Lord, that Your love for us is unconditional, and that You free us from any pressure to be thin, while also freeing us to be responsible and accountable for what we're eating and how we're caring for our bodies. Thank you, Lord, that I'm finally free to be me, and that at any size I can live a new lifestyle, an all-new free-to-be-thin lifestyle. In Jesus' name, Amen.

Appendix A

Free to Be Thin
"Food Supplements"

The following "Food Supplements" are passages of Scripture paraphrased as first-person statements to motivate and encourage you, and to help you apply the truth of Scripture to your daily experiences.

My old unrenewed self was nailed to the cross with Jesus. My body has been made ineffective and inactive for evil. I am no longer the slave of my fleshly appetites. I have died with Christ, and I also live with Him.   Based on Romans 6:6–8

I do not eat for reward.
I do not need such rewards.
I have my reward!
I have holiness and eternal life.   Based on Romans 6:22

I surrender and yield my appetite as an instrument of obedience to the Lord. I do not surrender to the demands of the flesh. I choose to be obedient to the Word of God. I crucify the flesh. I do not yield to the passions of the flesh. The flesh is dead.
Based on Romans 6:13–16

I do not let sin rule as king in my body to make me yield to its cravings. I am not subject to its lusts and evil passions. I do not offer or yield my bodily members to overeating but offer and yield myself to God. I have been raised from deadly habits to perpetual life. I present my body and its members to God as implements of righteousness.   Based on Romans 6:12–13

I do not surrender to temptations of the flesh, for I am not, nor will I become, a slave to the flesh. Rather, I choose to obey God.

I choose the way of righteous obedience. Here I am, Father; what would you have me do?   Based on Romans 6:16

I am a debtor, but not to the flesh. I am not obligated to my carnal nature—to live a life ruled by the standards set up by the dictates of the flesh—because if I live by the dictates of the flesh, I will surely die. But if by the power of the Holy Spirit I am habitually putting to death the deeds prompted by the body, I will really live forever.   Based on Romans 8:12–13

I consider that the sufferings of this present time are not worth being compared with the glory that is to be revealed to me and in me and for me and to be conferred on me.
                    Based on Romans 8:18

Who (or what) shall ever separate me from Christ's love? Shall suffering and affliction and tribulation? Or calamity and distress? Or persecution or hunger or destitution or peril or sword? It is for His sake I am put to death all day long. Yet amid all these things I am more than a conqueror and gain a surpassing victory through Him who loved me.   Based on Romans 8:34–37

I believe in You, Jesus.
    I trust You. I rely on You.
        I will not be put to shame, I will not be disappointed
            in my hopes, when they are centered in You.
                    Based on Romans 9:33

I am now experiencing steadfast patience and endurance and I am able to perform and fully accomplish the will of God. I receive and carry away and enjoy to the full what is promised.
                    Based on Hebrews 10:35–36

My way is not of those who draw back to eternal misery and are destroyed. But I am of those who believe. I cleave to and trust in and rely on God, through faith in Jesus Christ. By faith my soul is preserved.   Based on Hebrews 10:39

I choose at all times and for everything to give thanks in the name of my Lord, Jesus Christ, to God the Father.
                    Based on Ephesians 5:20

I put on God's whole armor. I have the armor of a heavily armed soldier; God has issued it to me. I am able to stand up successfully against all the strategies and the deceits of the devil.

Based on Ephesians 6:11

I choose to behave in faith and by practice of patient endurance and waiting, and I am now inheriting the promises.

Based on Hebrews 6:12

Since I have put on God's complete armor, I am able to resist and stand my ground on the evil day of danger. Having done all the crisis demands, I stand firmly in my place.

Based on Ephesians 6:13

It is impossible for God ever to prove false or deceive me. I have fled to Him for refuge, so that I might have indwelling strength and strong encouragement to grasp and hold fast the hope appointed for me.

Based on Hebrews 6:18

I have hope as a sure and steadfast anchor of my soul. It cannot slip and it cannot break away from me as I rely on God.

Based on Hebrews 6:19

I now seize and hold fast and retain without wavering the hope I cherish and confess. I acknowledge my goal of living a controlled and Free-to-Be-Thin lifestyle. God, who promised me His help, is reliable, sure, and faithful to His word.

Based on Hebrews 10:23

Appendix B

Questionnaire

Part One

1. What is your age? _____
2. Are you overweight now? _____
3. How much? _____
4. How long have you been overweight? _____
5. List your overweight relatives: _____
   _____
6. Have you been on a weight-loss program other than Overeaters Victorious before? _____
7. How many? _____
8. Have you ever been in Overeaters Victorious before? _____
   _____
9. What is the longest you have been able to maintain a weight loss? _____
10. Do you exercise regularly? _____
11. What kind of exercise do you like the most? _____
    _____
12. What kind of exercise do you like the least? _____
    _____
13. What are your hobbies? _____
    _____
14. Can you associate any kind of trauma or major life change with the onset of your weight problem? _____
    Explain: _____
    _____
15. How do you handle emergencies? _____
    _____

PART TWO

Briefly describe how you cope with

insecurity _____

_____

jealousy _____

_____

worry _____

_____

anger _____

_____

money problems _____

_____

fear _____

_____

joy _____

_____

put-downs by people you love _____

_____

rejection _____

_____

stress _____

_____

death of family member or friend _____

_____

grief _____

_____

sad feelings _____

_____

guilt _____

_____

sudden remembrance of painful memories _____

_____

PART THREE

Answer the following only if you are married:
1. Were you overweight when you got married? _____
2. If so, how much? _____
3. Was your weight a problem to your spouse then? _____
4. Is your weight a problem to your spouse now? _____

Does your spouse (Answer yes or no.)
5. Tease you about your weight? _____
6. Pressure you about your weight? _____
7. Admire others that are thinner in a way that you think is intended to make you notice? _____
8. Offer you food that you should not eat while on a weight-loss program? _____
9. Offer you sympathy when you are discouraged? _____
10. Know about your true feelings? _____
11. Listen when you need to talk? _____
12. Demand that you fix food you cannot eat? _____
13. Stay with you during kitchen cleanup? _____
14. Understand you? _____
15. Really know you? _____
16. Walk or engage in other exercise with you? _____
17. Help with the children? _____
18. Share his or her feelings with you? _____
19. Hide things from you? _____
20. Eat after meals in front of you? _____
21. Eat food you cannot have in front of you? _____
22. Treat you as an equal? _____
23. Love you? _____
24. Verbally express affection to you? _____
25. Support your participation in this study? _____
26. Based on the answers given above, would you say your spouse will be a support for you during this study? _____
    Explain. _____
    _____

QUESTIONS FOR CONSIDERATION

Please read each question carefully, then answer yes or no in column A. At the end of this study, answer the questions again (except for questions 1 and 22), using column B. Then compare your two sets of answers.

Question: A   B

1. Are you willing to weigh once at the beginning of this study and then not again until you have been prepared by the lessons?

2. Are you willing to eat only when sitting down, at a table, at meal times?

3. Are you willing to be accountable for every bite you eat?

4. Are you willing to use only one source for nutritional information, for calorie amounts, fat gram amounts?

5. Are you willing to incorporate exercise into your daily routine?

6. Are you willing to include your spouse (or other adults living with you) in your efforts to change your eating and exercise habits?

7. Are you willing to give up diet products?

8. Are you willing to drink more water?

9. Are you willing to live with the discomfort change can bring?

10. Are you willing to sacrifice, if necessary?

11. Are you willing to plan for and develop the habit of a daily quiet time?

	A	B

12. Are you willing to grocery shop with a list and stick to it?

13. Are you willing to put tempting foods out of the house or at least out of sight?

14. Are you willing to serve directly from the pans on the stove, putting only correct portions on your plate?

15. Are you willing to give up using food as a reward?

16. Are you willing to avoid using a slip as an excuse for a landslide?

17. Are you willing to learn to cook differently?

18. Are you willing to delay eating, when tempted, by calling your prayer partner for support?

19. Are you willing to face the fact that life will not be perfect simply because you are losing weight?

20. Are you willing to face the fact that you will from now on, for the rest of your life, have to change your eating habits to secure a Free-to-Be-Thin lifestyle?

21. Are you willing to face the fact that life will not be perfect when you are thin, simply because you are thin?

22. Are you willing to make every effort to attend this class session each week (or complete the course in a disciplined, timely manner if you are working on your own)?

23. Are you willing to eat balanced meals, avoiding fad diets and quick-solution methods?

24. Are you willing for your weight loss to take a long time, even while you're doing everything according to the guidelines?

APPENDIX D

A PROMISE TO MY OV PARTNER

You are my friend and I love you. I realize that you have allowed me to enter a very personal part of your life and that our relationship is special. I want you to know that I will endeavor to hold this trust according to the Word of God.

When you are down, I promise to try to help you up again. If I have fallen, too, and cannot pull you up with my own encouragement, I will still support you in prayer. I will provide warmth from the living Word of God when I sense you are growing cold. I will help you when you are weak.

I promise to be consistent in my support of you. I will not binge with you one day, then correct you for wanting to binge the next. If you want to binge, don't ask me to be a part of it. I will not tempt you in any way with food that is not on your program or in your best interest. Don't expect any fattening goodies from me.

If you should fail, I will be there to help you up and to lead you to the forgiving Savior.

I will endeavor to avoid being a stumbling block to you. I love you as I love myself. I want only your success. I will give others a good report of your work and the victory I see ahead for you.

I promise to bring you daily to the Father through prayer. I am confident of the work He is doing in you and that He will continue it in you until you reach the perfected image of His Son Jesus. I will keep a special place in my heart for you at all times.

I will keep you in mind when I am tempted to give up, realizing that my success is important to you. When I want to cheat or discard my planned food choices, I will remember that my diligence will help you be diligent, too.

When you need me to be firm, I will be firm. But I will always endeavor to be compassionate, patient, and gentle in our confrontations. What's more, I ask the same of you.

I will be sharing with you new truths and insights from the

Word of God as I am enlightened by the Holy Spirit. I will share with you the joy of discovering the living Christ through the Word.

I will seek creative ways to build you up in faith and to encourage you. I always want to seek the good in and for you.

I choose to accompany my faith for your success with works that enforce and confirm that faith. Don't expect me to feel your self-pity (should there be any) or to feel sorry for you when you pass up a treat neither of us needs.

We will make it this time, my friend! You, me, and Jesus.

_____   _____

OV partner   *OV partner*

SCRIPTURE REFERENCES FOR THE PARTNER PROMISE:

Ecclesiastes 4:9–12—We need mutual support.

Acts 20:35—We must help the weak.

Romans 14:21—Don't do anything that will cause your partner to fall.

1 Corinthians 8:9–13—Be careful not to provide stumbling blocks.

Galatians 5:14—Love others as yourself.

Galatians 6:10—Do only good for each other.

Philippians 1:3–7—Pray for each other; be confident of the work going on not only in yourself, but in each other. Keep each other in your heart.

Colossians 3:13—Bear with each other.

Colossians 3:12—Be patient and gentle, and show compassion.

Colossians 3:16—Teach and admonish each other from God's Word with psalms, hymns, and spiritual songs.

1 Thessalonians 5:11—Build up and encourage each other.

1 Thessalonians 5:15—Always seek after what is good for each other.

James 2:14–18—Faith without works is dead.

FOOD EXCHANGES

Here are the food exchanges for your calorie needs as computed in Lesson Three:

FOOD CHOICES[1]

Each day you need to eat a variety of foods. Each person's daily calorie and nutritional needs are different. A licensed nutrition counselor or registered dietitian can help you work out how many choices from each food group are just right for you. By eating foods from each food group, you will meet your basic nutritional needs. For a healthy diet, each day you should have *at least* four choices from the starch/bread group; five meat or meat substitute choices; two vegetable choices; two fruit choices; two skim milk choices; and not more than three fat choices. These choices add up to about 1200 calories per day.

The foods listed in each group are just examples. Many others can be part of your daily meal plan.

Starch/Bread

Each of these equals one starch/bread choice (80 calories). You have _____ choices each day.

½ cup pasta or barley
⅓ cup rice or cooked dried beans and peas
1 small potato (or ½ cup mashed)
½ cup starchy vegetables (corn, peas, or winter squash)
1 slice bread or 1 roll
½ English muffin, bagel or hamburger/hot dog bun
½ cup cooked cereal
¾ cup dry cereal, unsweetened
4–6 crackers

---

[1]Copyright (c) 1986, ADA. Used by permission.

3 cups popcorn, unbuttered, not cooked in oil

Vegetables

Each of these equals one vegetable choice (25 calories). You have
_____ choices each day.

½ cup cooked vegetables
1 cup raw vegetables
½ cup tomato/vegetable juice

Milk

Each of these equals one milk choice. The calories vary for each
choice. You have _____ choices each day.
1 cup skim milk (90 calories)
1 cup lowfat milk (120 calories)
8-ounce carton plain lowfat yogurt (120 calories)

Meat and Meat Substitutes

You have _____ choices each day. Each of these equals
one meat choice (75 calories).
1 oz. cooked poultry, fish, or meat
¼ cup cottage cheese
¼ cup salmon or tuna, water packed
1 tablespoon peanut butter
1 egg (limit 3 per week)
1 oz. lowfat cheese, such as mozzarella, ricotta
Each of these equals two meat choices (150 calories)
1 small chicken leg or thigh
½ cup cottage cheese or tuna
Each of these equals three meat choices (225 calories).
1 small pork chop
1 small hamburger
cooked meat, about the size of a deck of cards
½ of a whole chicken breast
1 medium fish fillet

Fruit

Each of these equals one fruit choice (60 calories). You have
_____ choices each day.
1 fresh medium fruit

1 cup berries or melon
½ cup fruit, canned in juice or without sugar
½ cup fruit juice
¼ cup dried fruit

Fat

Each of these equals one fat choice (45 calories). You have
_____ choices each day.
    1 teaspoon margarine, oil, or mayonnaise
    2 teaspoons diet margarine or diet mayonnaise
    1 tablespoon salad dressing
    2 tablespoons reduced-calorie salad dressing

Your Food Choices

    Calories Each Day:* _____

---

*As computed in Lesson Three, pages 49–50.

CALORIC INTAKE AND EXCHANGES

BREAKFAST	1400	1600	1800	2000
Bread	2	2	3	3
Meat*	0–1	0–1	0–1	0–1
Fruit	1	1	1	1
Milk	1	1	1	1
Fat†	0–1	0–1	0–1	0–1

LUNCH				
Bread	2	3	3	3
Meat	2	3	3	3
Vegetable	1	1	1	1
Fruit	1	1	2	2
Milk	1	1	1	1
Fat	0–1	1	1	2

DINNER				
Bread	3	3	3	3
Meat	3	3	4	4
Vegetable	1	1	1	2
Fruit	1	1	1	2
Milk	1	1	1	1
Fat	0–1	1	1	2

TOTALS				
Bread	7	8	9	9
Meat	5	6	7	7
Vegetable	2	2	2	3
Fruit	3	3	4	5
Milk	3	3	3	3
Fat	0–3	2–3	2–3	4–5

---

*On days when one protein is used at breakfast, delete one serving of protein from dinner.

†Adjust fat servings per totals allowed each day.

APPENDIX F

MENU IDEAS[1]

The following menu ideas have been prepared by Lisa Harris, RD, a licensed Nutrition Consultant. While no recipes are provided, preparation ideas are included. We have looked for simplicity and practicality in our menus.

Most of the items suggested are commercially available. Every nutritional standard is met and variety is encouraged. The calorie amounts at the top of the meal lists are the whole-day allotments.

In preparation, remember to keep your fat content as low as possible, and try to adapt some of your family's favorite recipes so you can eat with them as well. Remember, if it's good for you, it's good for them.

When serving canned fruit, rinsing is recommended unless it comes packed in light syrup or in fruit juice.

Bon Appetit!

---

[1]Reprinted from *Overcoming the Dieting Dilemma*, Neva Coyle, Bethany House Publishers, 1991.

Breakfast	1400	1600	1800	2000
#1				
wheat-flake cereal	¾ c	¾ c	1½ c	1½ c
whole wheat toast	1 slice	1 slice	1 slice	1 slice
orange juice	½ c	½ c	½ c	½ c
milk, skim	1 c	1 c	1 c	1 c
margarine	1 tsp	1 tsp	1 tsp	1 tsp
#2				
oatmeal, cooked with 1 tsp brown sugar	1 c	1 c	1½ c	1½ c
raisins	2 tbsp	2 tbsp	2 tbsp	2 tbsp
milk, skim	1 c	1 c	1 c	1 c
#3				
whole wheat English muffin	1	1	1½	1½
peanut butter	1 tbsp	1 tbsp	1 tbsp	1 tbsp
sliced apple w/cinnamon	1	1	1	1
milk, skim	1 c	1 c	1 c	1 c
#4				
whole wheat English muffin	1	1	1½	1½
scrambled egg	1	1	1	1
apple juice	½ c	½ c	½ c	½ c
milk, skim	1 c	1 c	1 c	1 c
margarine	1 tsp	1 tsp	1 tsp	1 tsp
#5				
cold cereal	1½ c	1½ c	1½ c	1½ c
whole wheat toast	0	0	1 slice	1 slice
banana	½	½	½	½
milk, skim	1 c	1 c	1 c	1 c
margarine	0	0	1 tsp	1 tsp

#6

hot cereal, cooked	1 c	1 c	1 c	1 c
with 1 tsp sugar & cinnamon				
raisin toast, unfrosted	0	0	1 slice	1 slice
orange juice	½ c	½ c	½ c	½ c
milk, skim	1 c	1 c	1 c	1 c
margarine	0	0	1 tsp	1 tsp

#7

Grape Nuts™	6 tbsp	6 tbsp	6 tbsp	6 tbsp
raisin toast, unfrosted	0	0	1 slice	1 slice
banana	½	½	½	½
vanilla yogurt, nonfat	½ c	½ c	½ c	½ c
milk, skim	½ c	½ c	½ c	½ c
margarine	0	0	1 tsp	1 tsp

#8

French toast:	2 slices	2 slices	3 slices	3 slices
whole wheat bread dipped in mixture of				
egg	1	1	1	1
milk, skim	2 tbsp	2 tbsp	2 tbsp	2 tbsp
cinnamon,				
honey or syrup (optional)	1 tbsp	1 tbsp	1 tbsp	1 tbsp
applesauce	½ c	½ c	½ c	½ c
milk, skim	¾ c	¾ c	¾ c	¾ c

#9

homemade "Danish":				
English muffin	1	1	1½	1½
ricotta cheese	¼ c	¼ c	¼ c	¼ c
applesauce	½ c	½ c	½ c	½ c
(sprinkle w/cinnamon and heat in toaster oven until cheese				
is melted)				
milk, skim	1 c	1 c	1 c	1 c

#10

whole wheat toast	2 slices	2 slices	2 slices	2 slices
flake cereal	0	0	¾ c	¾ c
poached egg	1	1	1	1
pineapple juice	½ c	½ c	½ c	½ c
milk, skim	1 c	1 c	1 c	1 c
margarine	1 tsp	1 tsp	1 tsp	1 tsp

#11

waffle, 4½" square	2	2	3	3
syrup, optional	1 tbsp	1 tbsp	1 tbsp	1 tbsp
applesauce	½ c	½ c	½ c	½ c
milk, skim	1 c	1 c	1 c	1 c
margarine	1 tsp	1 tsp	1 tsp	1 tsp

#12

graham crackers, 2½" square	6 each	6 each	6 each	6 each
wheat-flake cereal	0	0	¾ c	¾ c
cottage cheese, lowfat	¼ c	¼ c	¼ c	¼ c
cantaloupe	⅓ melon	⅓ melon	⅓ melon	⅓ melon
milk, skim	1 c	1 c	1 c	1 c

#13

muffin, oat bran or fruit	1 med	1 med	1 lg	1 lg
banana	½	½	½	½
milk, skim	1 c	1 c	1 c	1 c

#14

breakfast bar*, no more than 150 calories and 30% fat	1	1	2	2
apple juice	½ c	½ c	½ c	½ c
milk, skim	1 c	1 c	1 c	1 c

#15

instant breakfast mix* with skim milk	1 c	1 c	1 c	1 c
banana	½	½	½	½
whole wheat toast	0	0	1	1
margarine	0	0	1 tsp	1 tsp

---

*Commercial products found in the breakfast food section of the supermarket.

Lunch	1400	1600	1800	2000

#1

tuna sandwich with:

	1400	1600	1800	2000
whole wheat bread	2 slices	2 slices	2 slices	2 slices
tuna, water-packed	½ c	¾ c	¾ c	¾ c
mayonnaise, reduced calorie,	1 tbsp	1 tbsp	1 tbsp	2 tbsp
chopped celery and onions				
whole wheat crackers, no fat added	0	3	3	3
celery sticks	½ c	½ c	½ c	½ c
apple	1 small	1 small	1 large	1 large
milk, skim	1 c	1 c	1 c	1 c

#2

	1400	1600	1800	2000
chili with beans	1 c	1 c	1 c	1 c
grated lowfat cheese	0	1 oz	1 oz	1 oz
whole wheat roll	0	1	1	1
carrot sticks	½ c	½ c	½ c	½ c
banana	½	½	1	1
milk, skim	1 c	1 c	1 c	1 c

#3

	1400	1600	1800	2000
whole wheat pita with	1	1	1	1
turkey, chopped	2 oz	3 oz	3 oz	3 oz
lettuce	1 leaf	1 leaf	1 leaf	1 leaf
raisins	0	0	2 tbsp	2 tbsp
mayo, reduced calorie	1 tbsp	1 tbsp	1 tbsp	2 tbsp
grapes	15	15	15	15
animal crackers	0	8	8	8
milk, skim	1 c	1 c	1 c	1 c

#4

submarine sandwich:

	1400	1600	1800	2000
small roll	1	1	1	1
beef, lean	½ oz	½ oz	½ oz	½ oz
turkey	½ oz	1 oz	1 oz	1 oz
ham, lean	½ oz	1 oz	1 oz	1 oz
cheese	½ oz	½ oz	½ oz	½ oz
(slice meats and cheese very thin)				
mayo, reduced calorie	1 tbsp	1 tbsp	1 tbsp	1 tbsp

avocado	0	0	0	⅛
mustard				
pretzels	0	¾ oz	¾ oz	¾ oz
carrot sticks	½ c	½ c	½ c	½ c
orange, sliced	1	1	1	1
apple, sliced	0	0	1	1
milk, skim	1 c	1 c	1 c	1 c

#5

bagel	1	1	1	1
fruit "ambrosia":				
lowfat cottage cheese	½ c	¾ c	¾ c	¾ c
lowfat yogurt,	¼ c	¼ c	¼ c	¼ c
fruit-flavored				
peaches, diced	¼ c	¼ c	½ c	½ c
topped with Grape Nuts™	0	3 tbsp	3 tbsp	3 tbsp
salad	½ c	½ c	½ c	½ c
diet salad dressing	2 tbsp	2 tbsp	2 tbsp	2 tbsp
milk, skim	1 c	1 c	1 c	1 c

#6

vegetable soup	1 c	1 c	1 c	1 c
chicken salad sandwich:				
whole wheat bread	1 slice	2 slices	2 slices	2 slices
chicken, chopped	2 oz	3 oz	3 oz	3 oz
diet salad dressing	2 tbsp	2 tbsp	2 tbsp	4 tbsp
tomato	2 slices	2 slices	2 slices	2 slices
lettuce	1 leaf	1 leaf	1 leaf	1 leaf
pear, fresh	1 small	1 small	1 large	1 large
milk, skim	1 c	1 c	1 c	1 c

#7

baked chicken	2 oz	3 oz	3 oz	3 oz
baked beans	½ c	½ c	½ c	½ c
salad	½ c	½ c	½ c	½ c
diet salad dressing	2 tbsp	2 tbsp	2 tbsp	2 tbsp
whole wheat roll	0	1	1	1
banana	½	½	1	1
milk, skim	1 c	1 c	1 c	1 c

margarine	0	1 tsp	1 tsp	1 tsp

#8

spaghetti (cooked)	1 c	1 c	1 c	1 c
with: meatballs	1 oz	2 oz	2 oz	2 oz
sauce	½ c	½ c	½ c	½ c
parmesan cheese	2 tbsp	2 tbsp	2 tbsp	2 tbsp
bread sticks, 4" long	0	2	2	2
spinach	½ c	½ c	½ c	½ c
applesauce	½ c	½ c	1 c	1 c
milk, skim	1 c	1 c	1 c	1 c
margarine	0	1 tsp	1 tsp	2 tsp

#9

baked potato	1 large	1 large	1 large	1 large
topped with				
taco-flavored beef	2 oz	2 oz	2 oz	2 oz
shredded lowfat cheese	0	1 oz	1 oz	1 oz
sour cream	0	2 tbsp	2 tbsp	2 tbsp
margarine	0	0	0	1 tsp
green beans	½ c	½ c	½ c	½ c
Rye-Krisp™	0	4	4	4
pineapple, canned	⅓ c	⅓ c	⅔ c	⅔ c
milk, skim	1 c	1 c	1 c	1 c

#10

hamburger patty	3 oz	3 oz	4 oz	4 oz
with cheese	0	1 oz	1 oz	1 oz
pickles, catsup, mustard				
French fries	0	10 each	10 each	10 each
salad	½ c	½ c	½ c	½ c
diet salad dressing	2 tbsp	2 tbsp	2 tbsp	2 tbsp
apple	1 small	1 small	1 large	1 large
milk, skim	1 c	1 c	1 c	1 c

#11

cheese pizza	1 slice	1 slice	2 slices	2 slices
¼ of a 10" pizza				
with lean Canadian bacon	1 oz	2 oz	1 oz	1 oz
bread sticks, 4" long	0	2	1	1

salad	½ c	½ c	½ c	½ c
diet salad dressing	2 tbsp	2 tbsp	2 tbsp	2 tbsp
peach, fresh	1 small	1 small	1 large	1 large
milk, skim	1 c	1 c	½ c	½ c

#12
peanut butter & jelly
sandwich:

whole wheat bread	2 slices	2 slices	2 slices	2 slices
peanut butter	2 tbsp	2 tbsp	2 tbsp	2 tbsp
jelly	1 tbsp	1 tbsp	1 tbsp	1 tbsp
string cheese	0	1 oz	1 oz	1 oz
yogurt, lemon-flavored, nonfat	1 c	1 c	1 c	1 c
carrot sticks	½ c	½ c	½ c	½ c
graham crackers	0	3	3	3
apple juice	½ c	½ c	1 c	1 c
olives	0	5 large	5 large	10 large

#13
soft taco with

ground beef, lean	2 oz	2 oz	2 oz	2 oz
grated cheese	0	1 oz	1 oz	1 oz
lettuce & tomato	½ c	½ c	½ c	½ c
flour tortilla	1	1	1	1
refried beans	⅓ c	⅔ c	⅔ c	⅔ c
pears, canned	2 halves	2 halves	4 halves	4 halves
milk, skim	1 c	1 c	1 c	1 c

#14

frozen lowfat dinner (less than 300 calories)	1	1	1	1
salad	½ c	½ c	½ c	½ c
diet salad dressing	2 tbsp	2 tbsp	2 tbsp	2 tbsp
apple, sliced	0	0	1	1
milk, skim	1 c	1 c	1 c	1 c
(save for snack:)				
cheese	0	1 oz	1 oz	1 oz
saltines	0	6	6	6

Dinner	1400	1600	1800	2000
#1				
savory chicken breast	3 oz	3 oz	4 oz	4 oz
(marinate in low-cal Italian dressing)				
wild rice, cooked	⅔ c	⅔ c	⅔ c	⅔ c
whole wheat roll	1 small	1 small	1 small	1 small
broccoli	½ c	½ c	½ c	1 c
peaches, canned	½ c	½ c	½ c	1 c
milk, skim	1 c	1 c	1 c	1 c
margarine	1 tsp	1 tsp	1 tsp	2 tsp
#2				
baked halibut w/lemon	3 oz	3 oz	4 oz	4 oz
new potatoes	6 oz	6 oz	6 oz	6 oz
cooked w/parsley and				
margarine	1 tsp	1 tsp	1 tsp	2 tsp
baked beans	¼ c	¼ c	¼ c	¼ c
salad	½ c	½ c	½ c	1 c
diet salad dressing	2 tbsp	2 tbsp	2 tbsp	2 tbsp
fruit cocktail	½ c	½ c	½ c	1 c
milk, skim	1 c	1 c	1 c	1 c
#3				
spaghetti (cooked)	1 c	1 c	1 c	1 c
with				
ground beef	2 oz	2 oz	2 oz	2 oz
sauce	½ c	½ c	½ c	½ c
parmesan cheese	2 tbsp	2 tbsp	4 tbsp	4 tbsp
French bread	1 slice	1 slice	1 slice	1 slice
zucchini	½ c	½ c	½ c	1 c
frozen grapes	15 small	15 small	15 small	15 small
honeydew melon	0	0	0	1 c
milk, skim	1 c	1 c	1 c	1 c
margarine	1 tsp	1 tsp	1 tsp	2 tsp
#4				
BBQ flank steak	3 oz	3 oz	4 oz	4 oz
corn on the cob, 6"	1	1	1	1
noodles, cooked	1 c	1 c	1 c	1 c
seasoned w/parsley				
& margarine	1 tsp	1 tsp	1 tsp	2 tsp

green beans	½ c	½ c	½ c	1 c
strawberries	1¼ c	1¼ c	1¼ c	1¼ c
kiwi, slices	0	0	0	1
milk, skim	1 c	1 c	1 c	1 c

#5
Italian chicken:

breast	3 oz	3 oz	4 oz	4 oz
cooked in stewed	½ c	½ c	½ c	1 c
tomatoes				

(seasoned w/Italian seasoning, garlic & onion powder)

shell pasta, cooked	1 c	1 c	1 c	1 c
peas	½ c	½ c	½ c	½ c
apple, sliced	1	1	1	1
orange, sliced	0	0	0	1
milk, skim	1 c	1 c	1 c	1 c
margarine	1 tsp	1 tsp	1 tsp	2 tsp

#6

turkey, sliced	3 oz	3 oz	4 oz	4 oz
dressing	½ c	½ c	½ c	½ c
yams	⅓ c	⅓ c	⅓ c	⅓ c
green beans	½ c	½ c	½ c	1 c
applesauce w/cinnamon	½ c	½ c	½ c	1 c
milk, skim	1 c	1 c	1 c	1 c
margarine	0	0	0	1 tsp

#7

shrimp, steamed	6 oz	6 oz	8 oz	8 oz
black beans, cooked	⅓ c	⅓ c	⅓ c	⅓ c
(seasoned w/onions, garlic powder, mushrooms)				
brown rice, cooked	⅔ c	⅔ c	⅔ c	⅔ c
sliced tomatoes	3 slices	3 slices	3 slices	6 slices
diet gelatin w/ diced pears	½ c	½ c	½ c	1 c
milk, skim	1 c	1 c	1 c	1 c

margarine	1 tsp	1 tsp	1 tsp	2 tsp

#8

pork chops, broiled (trim fat)	3 oz	3 oz	4 oz	4 oz
potatoes, mashed	½ c	½ c	½ c	½ c
dinner roll	1 large	1 large	1 large	1 large
spinach	½ c	½ c	½ c	1 c
applesauce	½ c	½ c	½ c	½ c
w/raisins	0	0	0	2 tbsp
milk, skim	1 c	1 c	1 c	1 c
margarine	1 tsp	1 tsp	1 tsp	2 tsp

#9

beef stew (make in crock pot with no added fat)				
lean beef	3 oz	3 oz	4 oz	4 oz
potatoes, chopped	1 small	1 small	1 small	1 small
carrots	½ c	½ c	½ c	½ c
peas	½ c	½ c	½ c	½ c
biscuit	1	1	1	1
peaches, canned	2 halves	2 halves	2 halves	4 halves
milk, skim	1 c	1 c	1 c	1 c
margarine	0	0	0	1 tsp

#10

ham, lean	3 oz	3 oz	4 oz	4 oz
cornbread, 2" sq.	1	1	1	1
sweet potato	⅔ c	⅔ c	⅔ c	⅔ c
salad	½ c	½ c	½ c	1 c
diet salad dressing	2 tbsp	2 tbsp	2 tbsp	2 tbsp
fruit cocktail	½ c	½ c	½ c	1 c
milk, skim	1 c	1 c	1 c	1 c
margarine	0	0	0	1 tsp

#11

broiled swordfish	3 oz	3 oz	4 oz	4 oz
baked potato	1 large	1 large	1 large	1 large
w/chives & sour cream	2 tbsp	2 tbsp	2 tbsp	2 tbsp
salad	½ c	½ c	½ c	1 c
diet salad dressing	2 tbsp	2 tbsp	2 tbsp	2 tbsp
sherbet	¼ c	¼ c	¼ c	¼ c

raspberries	½ c	½ c	½ c	1 c
(save for snack:)				
banana	¼	¼	¼	½
milk, skim	1 c	1 c	1 c	1 c

#12

hamburger patty	3 oz	3 oz	4 oz	4 oz
whole wheat bun	1	1	1	1
lettuce & tomato,				
reduced-calorie	1 tbsp	1 tbsp	1 tbsp	2 tbsp
mayo				
mustard & catsup				
baked beans	¼ c	¼ c	¼ c	¼ c
watermelon cubes	1¼ c	1¼ c	1¼ c	1¼ c
cantaloupe	0	0	0	⅓ melon
milk, skim	1 c	1 c	1 c	1 c

#13

filet of sole, broiled,	3 oz	3 oz	4 oz	4 oz
with lemon & herbs				
baked potato (wedges)	1 small	1 small	1 small	1 small
broccoli	½ c	½ c	½ c	1 c
peach slices	½ c	½ c	½ c	1 c
milk, skim	1 c	1 c	1 c	1 c
margarine	1 tsp	1 tsp	1 tsp	2 tsp
angel food cake, ½ piece	1	1	1	1

#14

seasoned chicken, baked	3 oz	3 oz	4 oz	4 oz
w/choice of spices				
mashed potatoes	½ c	½ c	½ c	½ c
corn	½ c	½ c	½ c	½ c
salad	½ c	½ c	½ c	1 c
diet salad dressing	2 tbsp	2 tbsp	2 tbsp	2 tbsp
fruit cocktail	½ c	½ c	½ c	1 c
milk, skim	1 c	1 c	1 c	1 c
margarine	1 tsp	1 tsp	1 tsp	2 tsp
animal crackers	8	8	8	8

APPENDIX G

STEP-BY-STEP WALKING PROGRAM

Despite the great number of exercise programs that have been developed, many exercise experts still champion the benefits of walking. It's simple, it's safe, and it's long been proven effective. Walking not only contributes to cardiovascular health; it can also put you in a better mood!

All that's required for a good walking program is good walking shoes, loose, comfortable clothing, and your determination to do it regularly.

A good way to start is to plan your route ahead of time. Take your car and map out a two-mile course, as flat as possible for beginners, with a few slopes to be added later once you've been at it a while. Take it easy at first, pacing yourself so that if you were walking with a companion you could carry on a conversation without getting winded. Walk at least three (or better, four) days the first week. You might find your walk easier if you do a little stretching and bending before you go out. Take it easy—no pulled muscles, please!

After a week or two of walking with a leisurely stride, pick up the pace just a little so that you breathe a little harder, but still not so much that you couldn't carry on a conversation if you were walking with someone. If you're walking alone, try quoting a few favorite Scripture verses aloud to see if you can talk without being winded.

Time yourself: Is your speed two miles in thirty minutes? Next week try for two miles in 27 minutes and then two miles at 25 minutes. When you're walking two miles in 20 minutes, you'll know you're walking at a rate of 6 miles an hour. Eventually you'll want to increase your distance, and then begin to adjust your time again. When you're able, you'll find that a three-mile, thirty-minute walk is wonderful and beneficial. I guarantee you'll notice a difference the next time you're on a sight-seeing vacation—everyone will be trying to keep up with you!

Remember, the goal is to be fit, not fast! Fitness is a goal everyone at every weight can achieve. As our friend Stormie Omartian says, anything is better than nothing! Keep in mind that a walking program is built one step at a time. You must move step by step into health, step by step into fitness, step by step into your new lifestyle.

Chart your first few weeks here, recording the distance.

Miles and Minutes Walked				
Day:	1	2	3	4
Example:	2/40	2/40	2/42	2/38
Week One:				
Week Two:				
Week Three:				
Week Four:				
Week Five:				
Week Six:				